"A MUST-read before making a decision to have surgery. It may prevent surgery, or definitely reduce complications. Whether you need surgery or not, this book is a goldmine synthesizing the body-mind-emotions concepts that promote health and well-being.

It integrates the wisdoms and practices from my favorite holistic health professionals, and the sources cited are worth the cost of the book. By implementing the somatic practices, the concept of move it or loss with awareness, and the practical sense lifestyle suggestions, your health will improve. I only wish that I had read this book four years ago. It would have prevented my two-year recovery process following the complications from 'simple but botched' laparoscopic hernia operation."

—*Erik Peper, Ph.D., Professor of Holistic Health,
San Francisco State University, producer of the blog,
the peper perspective-ideas on illness, health
and well-being (www.peperperspective.com)*

"Noah Karrasch's book is a must-read for everyone to be better prepared for life's challenges, and the impact these challenges have both physically and mentally on our bodies. Noah's writing has your attention from the first to the last chapter. It is easy-to-read and understand, and packed with knowledge.

Having lived through emergency surgery and months of rehab due to a near-fatal automobile accident, I wish Noah's book, with all of the techniques he shares to speed up recovery, had been available to me then. Everyone should read and keep this book as their new go-to reference to healing their body!"

—*Deana L. Layton, Ed.D., educator and
survivor of near-fatal automobile accident*

"Years ago, I worked with an orthopedic surgeon who told me, 'There is no condition so bad that surgery cannot make it worse.' I did not know it at the time, but that wisdom would guide me through a long career in physical therapy. Noah's book nicely explains that surgeon's advice.

Find the right exercises and the right peace of mind. No matter your diagnosis, no matter your pain, if you want to understand how to best take care of your body, you need to read this book."

—*Bruce Linder, physical therapist*

"In today's world of over-prescribed everything—complete with a rising number of unnecessary surgeries—Noah's approach to healing is spot on. While he says, 'no one tool or practitioner is right for everyone, just as every tool or practitioner is right for someone', *The Self-Care Guide to Surgery* really does have something for everyone.

Ultimately, this book reminds us that when we take the time to stop and listen to our bodies, they will tell us what we need to know."

—*Gary Young, CNC, Zen Life Solutions*

"Yes, relax! As a (former) Type-A, tightly wound, often over-whelmed achiever, I have found Noah to be a true guide, and his emphasis on vagal health, relaxation and stress reduction to be literal lifesavers. I am healthier in so many ways because of his guidance.

The Self-Care Guide to Surgery is a great refresher, and not only helps people with significant health concerns, but also helps readers find balance and relax into their lives."

—Melissa Miller Young, Client

The Self-Care Guide to Surgery

by the same author

Meet Your Body
CORE Bodywork Tools to Release Bodymindcore Trauma
Noah Karrasch
Illustrated by Lovella Lindsey Norrell
ISBN 978 1 84819 016 0
eISBN 978 0 85701 000 1

BodyMindCORE Work for the Movement Therapist
Leading Clients to CORE Breath and Awareness
Noah Karrasch with Robert White and Elizabeth Buri
ISBN 978 1 84819 338 3
eISBN 978 0 85701 295 1

Getting Better at Getting People Better
Creating Successful Therapeutic Relationships
Noah Karrasch
ISBN 978 1 84819 239 3
eISBN 978 0 85701 186 2

Freeing Emotions and Energy Through Myofascial Release
Noah Karrasch
ISBN 978 1 84819 085 6
eISBN 978 0 85701 065 0

The
Self-Care Guide
to Surgery

A BodyMindCORE
Approach to Prevention,
Preparation and Recovery

Noah Karrasch

Illustrated by David Frizell

SINGING DRAGON
LONDON AND PHILADELPHIA

Disclaimer: The information contained in this book is not intended to replace the services of trained medical professionals or to be a substitute for medical advice. You are advised to consult a doctor on any matters relating to your health, and in particular on any matters that may require diagnosis or medical attention.

The poem on page 130 is reproduced with kind permission from Lucille Olson.

First published in 2020
by Singing Dragon
an imprint of Jessica Kingsley Publishers
73 Collier Street
London N1 9BE, UK
and
400 Market Street, Suite 400
Philadelphia, PA 19106, USA

www.singingdragon.com

Library of Congress Cataloging in Publication Data
A CIP catalog record for this book is available from the Library of Congress

British Library Cataloguing in Publication Data
A CIP catalogue record for this book is available from the British Library

ISBN 978 1 78775 167 5
eISBN 978 1 78775 168 2

Printed and bound in the United States

I'm old—yet
I'm vital—yet
I hurt much of the time—yet
It's a joy to keep moving.
Amen

Contents

Part II: Surgery!

Acknowledgments

Readers: Patricia Pike, Rupali Jeswal, MD, Roxanne Portman, Nanthakumar Kumaresan, Ralph Harvey, MD

Contributors: Daniel Kuebler, Ralph Harvey, MD

Illustrations: David Frizell

The doctors, nurses and staff of Mercy Hospital, Springfield, MO for care and lessons received

Friends, family and the support system that helps me to heal

Jessica Kingsley for tough questions, great ideas and constant encouragement

Disclaimer

I'm not a doctor! I'm a patient and a patient advocate. When in doubt, trust your doctor's advice, but never give up on seeking more information when you can't get the answers you need.

Prologue: Three Books in One

Why I'm Writing This Book...

It's said we all teach what we need to learn. For me, this has absolutely been true over the past 30-plus years as I've explored bodywork and health. Often a student would ask me to teach a subject and I'd feel inadequate, so I'd get to work and research and study. Sometimes I'd get interested in a subject because of my own body's challenges, or those of a client, and then I'd be off—researching, reading, thinking, practicing until I had a glimmer of the knowledge I felt needed to be shared. It's nearly always been the case, when I develop a new course for bodyworkers, that it's because I feel there's something I need to better understand so I can share it more clearly. I've written this book both to enhance my own knowledge of healing and to better share it with others who may need guidance on their potential or scheduled surgeries, or on how to heal from that which has already happened.

This book is anecdotal because it's full of what I know and how I've worked for many years, both with clients and with myself. I've had an interesting past with some spectacular and life-changing injuries. Mostly I allow myself to see them as teaching/learning experiences and try to grab as much of the useful knowledge from them as possible. In my recent past, working to be prepared for surgeries, then rehabilitating self after the traumas, has been an important goal and learning for me. I managed to keep an imminent surgery at bay for many years before finally giving in to the need for it, and I'm interested in sharing the "how" of that delay. Preventing, preparing for and rebuilding after surgeries has made me realize more and more that what I've learned in my own search could help others who face similar challenges. So, whether you're simply trying to live healthfully and thus avoid surgery, whether you're facing an upcoming surgery and want to be more fully prepared to minimize the pain and difficulty of the experience, or whether you've already had a surgery and are now trying to put life's pieces back together, I hope the ideas I share can help you manage your process on the road to potential surgery and recovery.

Some readers will discount the ideas I offer in this book because they could and will argue my claims aren't backed by research. While there's some truth to this claim, I do follow research, and am rather pleased to find much current research is pointing to the validity of many of my beliefs from the years of bodywork practice and observation of self and clients. A second point I'd argue: 34 years of doing bodywork has turned the anecdotes of the years into their own type of research. I watch what works and what doesn't; my own observations in my practice turn into recommendations for the most appropriate and efficient intervention if change is to happen. Anecdotes and hearsay have become an alternative research for me…just because I haven't documented along the way, or use no control groups, I don't think the results and learnings are less valid. Science and research are important, and I do pay attention, but I'm going to challenge you to use your own common sense instead of surrendering your authority to someone else. So even if these ideas seem a bit far-fetched or ungrounded to you, please give them serious consideration.

Along with my use of anecdotes in addition to research, I'm asking my friend Daniel Kuebler to share his surgery story as we work through the book. In the prevention, preparation and repair sections, Dan will talk briefly about what he did right and wrong, and how he's coping with decisions good and bad. We all make choices; sometimes we make right choices, sometimes we make learning opportunity choices. Dan and I have done both in our processes, and we hope to share some of our learning opportunities so you don't have to experience them for yourself.

I've also asked my brother-in-law of 30 years, Ralph Harvey, MD, to offer his perspectives as we reach the end of those chapters on prevention, preparation and repair. Ralph and I have considered ourselves colleagues in healing over the years, and each of us nudges the other to open the mind and discover new perspectives. I feel he's doing that for this book as well, and I'm delighted to have a medical doctor's take on my ideas.

The overriding concept and message of the book is simple: The more you take care of yourself, assume responsibility, seek good advice, make your own decisions and pay attention to your process, the better your chances are to not have a surgery, but also to be better prepared if one comes *and* to rehabilitate and repair yourself from a surgery more fully with the help of the ideas I share. You can achieve better health, at any stage along the journey, with thought, effort, commitment and intention.

Besides Common Sense, My Qualifications

As is true of so much of life, our largest challenges can be our greatest gifts and learning experiences. Surviving a crash landing of a small airplane in 1987 absolutely rocked my world, causing me to wonder if I'd walk again and whether my head would ever stop hurting, or whether I'd ever stop tasting blood when I touched my forehead. I've had a long journey of rehabilitation. I'm happy to say I've managed to recover most of my body from this early insult, back at age 37. Yet clearly at 69 I have more learning to do!

In the wreck my first lumbar vertebra was compression fractured (think both compressed and broken into many pieces) and was, in fact, so compromised that after the wreck my spinal column was squeezed into only 10 percent of the volume it should occupy. Sadly, this first lumbar vertebra is the most critical spot to have such an injury; one finds a bit of tissue in this area called *cauda equina* or "horse's tail." In this lower area of the spinal column the nerves split off into many different directions and functions in the lower body. Not knowing how this area would respond to time and treatment meant I might or might not regain the use of my left leg, of my bowels, of my bladder or of my sexual function.

> As is true of so much of life, our largest challenges can be our greatest gifts and learning experiences.

Happily, most of these functions have come back, though with quite a bit of work on my part, with some pieces still missing. For years bowel function has been slow moving, and I've had to work to manage the colon. In November of 2016, after 29 years of such management (and interestingly, one month after my first ever colonoscopy) my colon finally wore out, my stomach was in tremendous pain, and I sought help.

Something was happening in my body that I couldn't explain, and it was time to seek emergency guidance. After a CT scan, I was visited by an emergency room doctor who told me I had a perforated colon and that I'd soon be having surgery to remove the perforated section, staple the lower and upper parts of that removal shut, and cut a hole in my abdominal wall through which my bowel movements would occur for the foreseeable future, and perhaps forever. That's quite a difficult pill to swallow! Yet, what were my options?

Since severely breaking my back in that plane wreck 30 years before, my elimination system has been slow and problematic. Finally, the body said "no more" and I had to accept medical intervention. I was devastated, but as I'd managed to live an extra 30 years without surgery, and as I could tell that colon function had become more difficult, I knew it was time. Surgery was upon me, so I said yes.

"We'll remove a seven-inch section of perforated colon; we'll shut off your colon for now and give you a colostomy. You'll have bowel movements through this hole in the abdomen until you decide whether to have a reconstructive surgery in the future, perhaps six months after this initial operation." In a state of extreme pain, one tends to listen to the doctor, forget to ask questions and say yes to whatever can help alleviate pain! That very day I had a colostomy surgery. Afterwards, in addition to incredible stomach pain, I had to learn to deal with bowel movements erupting from a hole in my abdomen—on their own erratic schedule. As I was able to "train" my colon to produce its main release in the early morning hours, I managed to live a fairly normal life. However, I wanted the freedom to not have this system in my stomach, so six months later I met with the doctor to discuss the surgery to reconstruct my colon, what is commonly called a "colostomy takedown."

Retrospectively, I did several things wrong in my own preparation/rehabilitation cycle for this so-called "takedown" surgery, as I think many of us do. I'd done well in that six-month gap between the two surgeries, but, when the time came for actual surgery, I wasn't as ready as I thought. Though I'd studied and researched after the colostomy surgery to find out what the reversal procedure entailed, I didn't think to ask some of the appropriate questions for this one…questions that would have saved me heartache when expectations of healing weren't fulfilled in a timely fashion. While I didn't trust my gut reaction to the surgeon the first time I met him (and that gut knowledge was eventually borne out), with some hard work I feel reasonably healthy again. I'm not completely there, but the knowledge I've garnered has helped me grow, and, I think, could help lots of people in this and similar situations by providing insights and warnings as to what works and what doesn't.

I won't pretend I'm totally "back" from my surgeries; on the other hand, I'm not dead, and have had a pretty good life for the past 30 years! So, I tend to focus on the gratitude of having not only survived the traumas, but of having been given extra years to live and grow and take care of myself and regain my body. And, sometimes, I believe we must make peace and live with "where we are" with gratitude instead of yearning for more.

I don't see anything wrong with wanting more; I also don't see the value in wishing life was better without taking some action and movement towards that better life. Either we're taking positive steps, negative steps or staying still. Where are you? I hope you'll see the value of taking care of self, before, during and after any potential surgery.

How to Use This Book

So: I'm writing what I hope will be an informative book, in some ways three separate books. The first part of this book, *Balance in All Things*, is general common sense that hopes to nudge you into slowing down a hectic and unhealthy lifestyle, paying attention to your bodymindcore, taking a bit more responsibility for your health and considering ideas that can help you stay healthy, wherever you find yourself on the spectrum from vital to very ill. We'll look at five major components or qualities of successful living, based on my model of body centers that want and need to be in balance. Each supports and intersects with the others. If you can find and keep the balance of honoring each of these five areas I think you'll live a healthier life and, with luck, never need that surgery!

The five elements I'm offering that want balance to create a healthy body focus on the four centers of the body I'm most interested in keeping open and energetic: the head, heart, gut and groin. In addition to those four centers, our major building blocks, I'm adding a fifth area of the body to consider: the extremities. Though arms and legs clearly initiate from the four centers, in some ways they are their own entities and deserve to be examined separately. We'll discuss each of these five areas and focus on ways to keep open energetic channels moving through the body centers and to the extremities, through healthy thoughts (head), healthy breath and circulation (heart), healthy nutrition (gut), healthy survival, social connectedness and safety (groin) and healthy movement (extremities). When all these aspects are in balance and working together, we become and remain healthy beings. When these aspects are out of balance or underused, we lose our precious health.

In the past year I've realized most alternative practitioners focus on the restoration of energetic movement through the body. Yet too many medical personnel are interested in *stopping or slowing* that flow of energy, in their desire to alleviate or even destroy symptoms that tell us something is wrong with the body. Which model makes sense to you?

After the Extremities chapter of this first part, we introduce Chapter 6, an important idea and a small booklet of its own, what I think of as *Mindful Movement, Where You Are*. It's my concept that movement is critical to health and, as most of us won't move often enough, we're stagnating. As we discuss the extremities of the body, we'll spend far more time with the concept of getting our bodies out of the chair and into the world…reaching out to the world instead of shrinking from it.

Through the book, but especially in Chapter 6, I'll invite you to move more often and more forcefully…movement is critical to getting and staying healthy. Consider how stairs can be a good workout. Also, lifting ourselves in and out of an armchair, doing big toe pushups while cooking or washing and drying dishes, and shifting in the driver's seat or computer chair can all be seen as a dance and a simple way to bring movement back into our lives. I challenge all of us to be more fully involved in staying healthy by seeing everything around us as exercise and stretching equipment…be it your favorite armchair or recliner, the doorway you could push against as you go through or the trim above from which you can simply hang, or the counter or chair arms you could easily just put a little pressure onto and lift your body up and away from a bit more often. How can we move more freely and mindfully, right where we are, more of the time, instead of choosing to lock into a position, maintain it, stop breathing and begin hurting? I also include a *Quick Reference Guide* at the back of the book so you can find and return to any particular exercise you want to reclaim easily.

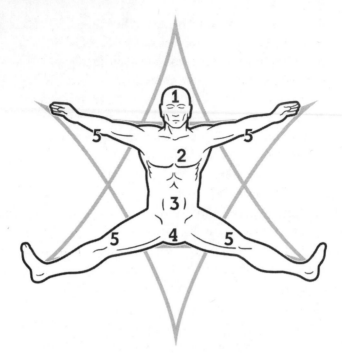

Four personal centers that require balance for a healthy
bodymindcore, plus the extremities that are guided by those centers.

I'm reminded of my initial meeting with C. Norman Shealy, MD, PhD, author, lecturer, thinker, neurosurgeon… Norm lives in my town, Springfield, Missouri. On moving to Springfield many years ago, I developed a network of health-oriented folk, and we gathered to attend a lecture by Norm at the institute where he was then teaching. I believe it was in this first lecture that I heard him use the image of your life's essence being held in a teacup, and your body being that cup. If each stressor in your life adds a bit more liquid, eventually, if you're adding stressors without ever pouring any of them out, you'll overflow. You'll become ill. Whether the cup is cracked, or whether it's simply overflowing with stress—either way, it's not healthy. If we can repair a crack in the body so we can hold more stress, that's fine. Doesn't it seem better both to introduce fewer stressors and to try to empty the cup more frequently?

Norm shared a stress test he used to help patients measure their own stress load and vulnerability. Among all the top stressors (divorce, death of loved one, major illness, birth of child, change of career/job, change of location, loss of old social support system) I was stunned to find I had somewhere around three times the acceptable level of stressors in my bodymindcore at that time! Oops…and interestingly, within a year I had my major challenge and a very major surgery—a plane wreck, a spinal fusion and seven-inch steel Harrington rods installed in my broken body.

Part II gives you as reader ideas and suggestions as to how you can do three things, depending on which part of the surgery spectrum you're now living: the first chapter of Part II,

Chapter 7, is devoted to positive actions you can take to prevent surgery. What lifestyle changes might you make to create a healthier you?

Chapter 8 will be the preparation phase: You've now discussed with a doctor that surgery's imminent. Perhaps you're in emergency mode and it's today; more likely this is something you've seen coming if you were paying attention. What steps can you take and what information can you gather before surgery comes, to enhance your healing and your ability to deal with the current or coming pain and trauma? What can you do to make your healing time after surgery shorter by preparing your body and yourself? There are options and tools to cut that recovery time down by giving attention to thoughtful preparation.

And in Chapter 9 we'll examine a critical question: How do we recover from such an insult, a trauma, an invasion? Many of us will feel totally bruised and beaten by our surgery. How do we get our movement, our appetite, our thoughts and our purpose back on track when we're so battered and bruised, so sore and sick? How do we give ourselves the time and space to heal and restore as we step back into our busy world? Perhaps most important, how do we make peace with and rejoice in what we still have instead of endlessly grieving for what we've lost?

Each of these segments—prevent, prepare and rebuild—will be grounded in general common-sense ideas. First among them: Relax! You can get through this. Whether you think you're ready for the changes coming, or whether you don't think you're ready, you're correct…so why not prepare mentally and physically to face the challenges ahead?

If you want to prepare for or cope with surgery, certainly jump ahead to "your" section of the book. Know that each chapter of the book contains information that will be helpful at any time, and that the first part offers good common sense whether you're healthy or not. In fact, no matter where you are on the spectrum, I'd recommend reading the entire book first, then going back to the specific area that's most needed by you right now. The ideas that help you recover from surgery more quickly may also help you prevent another as well.

And here's one more critical thought to consider as you work with this book: Figure out how to create and succeed with moderate, achievable goals instead of ambitious ones that may cause you to become discouraged and fail. Both kinds of goals are good; yet, at this time, moderating, achieving success and feeling even small progress will eventually accomplish more. Most important, it's easier to stay on the path if you don't push yourself so hard and fast towards achievement that you're doomed to fail. Give yourself some slack! I'll share later in another context that one of my favorite affirmations is "I am satisfied with my progress." Find one simple, daily activity involving breath and movement; start small but enhance that activity. Find your way to the whole you.

So let's begin! In that spirit, I offer ideas to help us live healthy, stay healthy, and prevent any necessary intervention by staying ahead of our bodies. Good luck on your journey!

Part I

BALANCE IN ALL THINGS

The Head: Healthy Thoughts Shape a Healthy World

First: Get your head on straight!

We often hear someone suggest "Her illness is all in her head." There may be more truth to that sentiment than we're ready to accept. In the past I've thought about two words: psychosomatic and somatopsychic (or a word bodyworker, author and educator Stanley Rosenberg used in *Accessing the Healing Power of the Vagus Nerve*,[1] somatopsychological). To me, psychosomatic suggests that, in fact, the head does affect how we feel, but somatopsychic suggests that, when we're in pain, it's hard to remain a rational being. Either condition contributes to feelings of illness and poor health.

How do we keep a "good head on our shoulders"? How do we find, develop and maintain a healthy life without overthinking the world or trying to avoid it? How does our brain create a life that's supportive, enthusiastic and affirms us and our worth, instead of knocking us down at every opportunity? It's so easy to spin our wheels, like a hamster in its cage, churning through life and its challenges instead of riding along as the wheel turns!

The brain is a marvelous organ, controlling both the nervous system which allows the body to function, but also

---

1   S. Rosenberg (2017) *Accessing the Healing Power of the Vagus Nerve.* Berkeley, CA: North Atlantic Books.

the endocrine system: that mechanism which tells the body how much of any chemical to release to keep balance throughout the being. While it can be argued (I believe correctly) that the brain is actually in every cell of the body, I see the head and its brain as the **control panel** of the body.

Many leaders in the alternative health community suggested illness is a form of meditation. That's rather a radical idea for some of us, but think of it: Have you ever found yourself with a cold just as you've come through a very trying and busy time? Can you see how your body might have been telling you it was tired and ready for the rest? Do you get sick when you feel overwhelmed? I remember the old joke: "As soon as the rush is over, I'm having a nervous breakdown...I've earned it and nobody can take it away from me!"

Let's visit the work of Dr. John Sarno. His book *The Divided Mind* suggests many of us suffer from what he calls tension myositis syndrome or TMS.[2] He believes most of us are in physical pain due to unexamined mental/emotional trauma; we'd rather let that pain manifest as body pain than sort through the emotional strain. His work gets people better if and when they realize that, in fact, they do stifle and don't process their emotions, and this self-censoring causes or contributes to their physical pain. Patients who can't understand or have faith in this model don't seem to get better from his work. Their pain is in their head, because they won't feel it in their bodies!

And let's introduce Peter Levine, author of *Waking the Tiger*[3] and founder of Somatic Experiencing technique, which encourages clients to revisit their traumas while paying attention to *body* sensations instead of focusing on their traumatized feelings. He's found that those who can stay anchored in exploring what the body tells them as they visit their trauma get well.

It's true the practitioner can push too hard and too fast, thus causing that trauma to get buried deeper. But the therapist

---

2   J. Sarno (2006) *The Divided Mind*. London: Harper.
3   P. Levine (1997) *Waking the Tiger*. Berkeley, CA: North Atlantic Books.

titrates (as in chemistry, we simply don't add too much stimulus at any one time to avoid the explosion or meltdown) the amount of work being done so clients can stay with their sensations. The therapist also *pendulates* and moves back and forth between the traumatic experience and a happier one that allows the body to return to calm. With a trained and compassionate therapist who follows these rules, keeping clients in their trauma space but focusing them on body sensations, they can get well. Levine and his followers are having great success dealing with clients who suffer with post-traumatic stress disorder or PTSD—a mental condition brought on by a mental or physical trauma.

So physical medicine doctor Sarno tells us we need to be more in touch with our emotions to release physical pain, while psychologist Levine suggests we tune into body sensations to release the emotional pain. I think both are right. And I'm reminded that John Pierrakos, developer of CORE Energetics and author of the book by the same name,[4] suggests we're three-layered beings. Pierrakos tells us our *core* is the Center Of Right Energy; our essence. He calls the *body* (the fascial network, which we'll discuss later) the second layer of our being, and our *environment* is the third layer. It's his contention that most of us use our brains to tighten our bodies to protect our cores from our environment. Does this idea ring true for you? Can you relax your body and enjoy your environment as you reach out to it? Or do you stay in protective mode, calling TMS to yourself?

Levine, Sarno and Pierrakos suggest we become healthier when we're able to allow the world and its traumas to move through us. Fear and anger seem most to slow this breeze of energy down in our bodymindcores. Can we allow ourselves to look our fear in the eye, to rise above it and grow anew? Can we find, face, feel and forget our fears and traumas which tighten our bodies all through our connective tissue network so arms and legs can't "express"?

---

4   J. Pierrakos (2005) *CORE Energetics*. Mendacino, CA: CORE Evolution.

I'll bring in another resource: Michael Harner studied shamanism around the world and realized that most shamanic cultures practice "soul retrieval." If this idea interests you, see Sandra Ingerman's book *Soul Retrieval: Healing the Fragmented Self*,[5] in which she describes Harner's work. The shaman or spirit-led healer goes into an altered state and finds and restores pieces of the ill person's soul; pieces that have been left in the past due to injuries or traumas. As s/he brings those soul's parts back together, the person often heals. It's an interesting thought which again invites us to do the work of facing the past and letting go of the hurts.

Henry Ford is reputed to have said "Whether you think you can or you think you can't, you're right." I agree...good health begins with a healthy head, a healthy mind. When our brain is too full of all the "what if" and "I should" and "if they really knew me" thoughts, how can we find time to enjoy our environment, as we work ever harder to protect our core? We've got to give our brains a rest!

I've thought about this for some time...there seems to be a new universal condition among too many of us. I'd name the condition "overwhelmed." I've watched television programs about hoarders and had a few among my family and friends. I've seen friends and clients depressed after the loss of a loved one or a special pet, or a major change in their circumstances that keeps them from their joy. I've witnessed people who feel financially buried, as if they're getting further behind every day. I've seen people who want to lose weight, quit smoking or drinking, or reconnect with loved ones from whom they've become estranged. In each case many of these folks can't get that first step made...or the second, or the third. I feel most of these conditions point to the feeling of being "overwhelmed" by something outside of ourselves. Ultimately, however, that which

5   S. Ingerman (2011) *Soul Retrieval: Healing the Fragmented Self.* New York: Harper One/Harper Collins.

is overwhelming us seems to be coming from inside instead. Truly, it is "all in our head."

Others can motivate us, but the best motivation is that which comes from inside us and whispers (sometimes shouts) to us that it's time to make changes. Most of us hear this voice, but many of us do everything we can to ignore and discount it. *So, the first step towards deciding to be healthier and happier is simply, take any step. Then give yourself credit for even the smallest effort.* Retrain your brain. Even if overwhelmed, one can set small goals and take small steps, celebrating tiny victories.

Many years ago I began my bodywork practice in a new town, freshly divorced, estranged from the community I'd built. Remember Dr. Shealy's stress test from the Prologue? Add depression to overstress, and you have a picture of me. Many days I'd go to my office with few or no clients on the books, lie down for a "quick" nap, and wake up an hour or two later, only to get up, use the toilet, then go back for another quick nap. It wasn't working, and I could tell because people were staying away in droves. I decided something had to change.

I began making short lists for each day. The list might be this simple:

- Go to the office.

- Wait for the mail.

- Make one or two phone calls to connect with past clients or reach out to a new one.

- Go out to lunch to be seen and possibly make a connection.

Creating smaller, more accomplishable goals instead of getting bogged down by that which was too hard worked for me; it helped to have a simple, achievable list. I didn't always complete all the two to four things on the list; sometimes one or even none was accomplished. But I tried to celebrate the few small victories I made. I didn't set huge unattainable goals, but I so enjoyed scratching off insignificant items. I didn't ask myself to overachieve; I just took tiny steps every day. And it worked. After a time, the few seeds I'd sown came to grow and clients began to come. I began to think and feel better about myself, which translated to a positive energy I could share with others, and they were attracted to me instead of wanting to get away from my depressed energy.

So how do you take those first tiny steps? The word that continues to come into my mind is "motivation." Take an action; any action that propels you towards something instead of away from the world and further into self and self-pity. Reprogram your brain. Create tiny achievable goals that allow you to feel a bit successful instead of constantly feeling like a failure. And don't expect someone else can do this work for you. We all look for that magic pill, that perfect panacea that will make things right in our world. For the most part the panacea comes from within once you've made steps towards finding it. If you never send your ship out, chances are it will never come in. It's up to you to get a good head on your shoulders! Remember, it all begins with one step, no matter how small.

The Science Is Clear

I've been studying the vagus nerve and its effects on health for several years and am convinced it's one of the brain's major pieces in the puzzle of optimal health and longevity. Possibly you've heard of the vagus nerve; probably you've heard of "fight or flight" syndrome. I think they're very much related.

The vagus is a fascinating piece of our body, and is beginning to get the respect it deserves, thanks in large part to Stephen Porges, author of *The Polyvagal Theory* and primary researcher of the vagus, and to psychologist Levine, author of the aforementioned *Waking the Tiger* and the more recent *In an Unspoken Voice.*[6] Recently I've found a new and important book by Stanley Rosenberg, rolfer, craniosacral therapist and educator. His previously mentioned *Accessing the Healing Power of the Vagus Nerve* seems to me to be the clearest explanation of exactly what and where the vagus is and what it does. It moves beyond other current writings to include relationships of other cranial nerves and the spinal column to this vagal complex. It also includes several easy recommendations for what I call the "reset" of the vagal system.

All these sources see the importance of vagal health to enhancing heart rate variability or HRV (an indicator of overall health; we'll return to it later), to breathing deeply and to letting go of stress and relaxing the entire bodymindcore. It's again common sense; when we get stressed, if we can remember to stop, take a few deep breaths and get on with our day, we'll be healthier and resilient more of the time. Remember how our elders used to encourage us to calm down and take a breath and we'd be fine? Intentional breath work can assist in that calming.

The vagus is the only one of the 12 cranial nerves to descend from the head into the body; the rest all remain in the head, enervating sight, smell, taste, equilibrium, and so on. Its name means "the wanderer" and it definitely does wander through the trunk of the body. Visualize the vagus as two upside down trees, left and right. They move next to the carotid artery channels at the side of the neck and down into the body where they divide into many branches. While the "roots" of this nerve are in the head, each of its body branches has a special function, providing the autonomic or automatic behavior to a particular organ or system. I consider the vagus to be the most important nerve of the body. Where some call it the "anti-anxiety nerve," I think of it as the nerve of well-being. When the vagal system

---

6   S. Porges (2011) *The Polyvagal Theory.* New York: W.W. Norton; P. Levine (1997) *Waking the Tiger* and (2010) *In an Unspoken Voice.* Berkeley, CA: North Atlantic Books.

can function well, we're calmer, more relaxed; when it's jangled, so are we.

As they've studied the nervous system, researchers find the vagus innervates autonomically all the organs and systems: stomach, heart, liver, lungs, kidneys; adrenal, reproductive, digestive, and eliminative systems, and so on. All these organs and systems are run by this vagal network in a backup or autonomic mode, through the brain's control panel. Another aspect of this autonomic system is found in the spinal nerves which move the sympathetic system, which we'll visit in a moment.

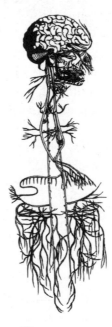

Vagus nerve.

When the system is overstimulated, we go into adrenal overload. And, thus, we're now into the endocrine system; that system of glands that regulates how the body works. The oldest response to this overload, the old mammal in us, wants to play dead. We *freeze*, somewhat like a possum would do when it senses danger. Second line of defense: the sympathetic nervous system in the spinal column thinks it must do something—action! It evaluates the situation and decides if it's wise to stand and *fight*. The body may decide to run away or *flee* instead.

So we have three separate coping paths to take when we sense danger: a too hot or cold room, an emotional outburst from a family member or colleague, a car nearly running us down, a missed appointment, a fall down the stairs—*anything* that pulls us off balance. The bodymindcore faces the situation and tries to shut down what it can, or move when it must do so, to cope with the threat. It automatically turns off unnecessary functions to deal with a situation in the moment. These functions hopefully come back online when the threat is past.

Fortunately, *and* unfortunately, we also have a parasympathetic system that corrects after that danger has passed… it suggests all is well and invites us to go back to our homeostasis, our "all systems operating smoothly" mode. This parasympathetic system gives us back what we're calling social engagement; it brings us back to reality and lets us know we can manage and are managing our reality. Sadly, too much of the time we seem to have gotten both sympathetic and parasympathetic stuck in "on" position. If the sympathetic system is the gas pedal that says, "get out of here, go!" and the parasympathetic is the brake or responder that says, "all clear now, chill," we unfortunately too often keep both pedals to the floor. Relax? I don't think so. So, how can we soothe this nervous system? Can you see why we're stressed, since our nervous system is overwhelming our brains?

Beth Spindler's book *Yoga Therapy for Fear*[7] suggests we could accurately describe these three states of fight, flee and freeze with simple words expressing how we behave in each situation: "blame, shame and should." When we fight, we blame: we look for ways to defend and make the "other" wrong.

---

7   B. Spindler (2018) *Yoga Therapy for Fear*. London and Philadelphia: Singing Dragon.

When we shame, we're overwhelmed by and run away from ourselves, our situations and our feelings. And when we freeze, we get stuck in our "shoulding" on ourselves; we can't decide how to improve our situation. How do we get away from these reactive solutions and back to parasympathetic function, shaking it out and moving on?

The newest part of this vagal system, evolution-wise, is the ventral vagus nerve. This is the "social engagement" system; the part of us that realizes there is a better solution to our problems than any of the actions the spinal sympathetic system or the dorsal vagus can provide. It's the myelinated or protein covered fibers that allow us to look at our world and *cope* with it.

I think of this position in the middle of a fight/flee/freeze triangle as the "find it/face it/feel it/forget it" mode. Porges identifies this protein-covered ventral vagus as giving us self-regulation and therefore social connectedness. I believe if and when we simply stop, breathe, examine, explore and, if necessary, *express* our feelings, we calm ourselves and return to the neutral, parasympathetic all-clear that allows us to move forward with life calmly and joyfully.

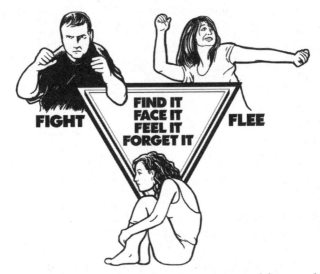

Many of us choose to default to and stay in one corner of the triangle, instead of staying in the central, feeling and self-regulation mode.

It's a fearful world these days! Between hurricanes, fires, volcanoes and other natural disasters, political upheavals, and economic and environmental problems, most of us are constantly in some form of fight/flee/freeze. Our brain is sadly overprogrammed to ACT, to move, to do something instead of to stop, to rest, to wait, and think, feel and process our questions and answers before we take action.

So, we're trying to learn to shake out our traumas as our animal friends can do. Think of a deer in the forest; imagine it hears a small noise. Immediately the deer will perk up, freeze, stare intently and listen to identify the danger. If it decides safety is critical, it may well bound away (flee). Rarely does it decide to fight, especially any unknown enemy such as a hunter. But if it decides the danger isn't there after all, it will make a brisk shake of the body before going back to whatever it was doing before the danger signal presented itself. Think of the possum that senses danger, and literally looks dead until something in its body suggests it's time to come back to the living. Sadly, many of us have forgotten that parasympathetic shake-it-out activity. We're stuck in adrenal overload, too often freezing (numbing out and playing dead, hoping the danger isn't interested in dead meat), fleeing (running away from a situation and observing from a distance) or fighting (digging in to stand our ground and achieve dominance). We could all profit from remembering to look back to the shake-it-out finding/feeling/facing/forgetting mode, instead of allowing ourselves to stay stuck in our default coping response. Our brains could profit from a simple house cleaning as we return to ventral vagus function and decide to "shake it out" and move on.

> I believe if and when we simply stop, breathe, examine, explore and, if necessary, express our feelings, we calm ourselves and return to the neutral, parasympathetic all-clear that allows us to move forward with life calmly and joyfully.

Too many of us return to those uncomfortable places where others abuse us, verbally, mentally, emotionally and sometimes even physically. We could learn to set boundaries that state, "I believe (and *feel*) I'm worth having around, and I'll interact with you unless you invalidate me. When I'm feeling discounted and disrespected, I can and will find a new environment where I can feel appreciated, loved, and respected." Can we search out people and situations that make us feel and accept positive touch, mental and physical? I've realized for some years now that we train people as to how we expect them to treat us…why would we train people to abuse us? Yet many of us do just that, discounting our own opinions and worth, focusing on giving but never receiving, or acting as a "punching bag" for those we "love." This is not self-nourishing.

Some of us just can't get to that space of nourishing our self. How do we become self-nurturers if it's opposite of everything we've learned about life to date? How can we make peace with where we are and be satisfied with our progress in more moments? If we're interested in better nutrition in every aspect of our life, what about our emotional nutrition? What are we feeding our brain? Mental preparation and self-acceptance are critical when you're ready to relate to others in a healthy fashion. How do you retrain yourself, especially if you've heard negativity from your friends, family or other support system in the past and present?

First, keep an attitude of gratitude. Give thanks: give thanks for the support system you have in place (even if it's small, find one!). Give thanks for the people who surround you and work with you—even if you must stretch the truth as you work to find the positive in them and the situations you share. Give thanks you have the stamina to say yes to activities or procedures that have you worried or challenged, then give thanks when you've succeeded in even a bit of those challenges.

Acknowledge your worries and fears. But choose to see that things can work out, and they possibly will, and work to remain positive and grateful. Find people who validate positive feelings. That's easy to say, and sometimes very difficult to do. But it's an attitude worth developing. Finding and maintaining a support system can feel like climbing a very high mountain; yet receiving support makes life so much better! Many of us will seek support but aren't ready to accept suggestions. Too many of us just want someone to "make it better"…yet most of us know the true healer lies within, and it's our responsibility to make life better ourselves. Easy to say, hard to do, because changing the world around us first requires change within, and most of us don't want it to work in that order. We want the world to change for us, *not* vice versa.

> I've realized for some years now that we train people as to how we expect them to treat us…why would we train people to abuse us?

After finishing this manuscript, I asked several friends to read and comment. A doctor in India points out just how hard it is to find and feel gratitude when one is far down. "Knowing and doing are two different things." She's right. We may know what's necessary, but it can take some real work to get our bodies to accept what our brain knows. When we're in the negative phase, our minds get clouded with blaming, it's hard to be accepting, and negative emotions take over. These negatives can be: *confusion* (run away?)—I don't understand how I got here and what I'm supposed to do to change; *repression* (play dead?)—If I pretend nothing is wrong, maybe it will go away; *feeling threatened* (fight back?)—I get angry and want to blame someone, because I'm scared and worried. If we can consciously examine these feelings, to *feel*, we can bring ourselves to adaptation and move through the negatives (stay present?)…*if* we make the effort, find support and stay positive about what we're achieving.

Many self-help programs deal with the need to face and process our fears and move forward in life. I've been involved in Twelve Step programs as a family member of an alcoholic, and through a prosperity program based on the twelve steps. I've participated in Steps Four and Five of the Twelve Steps on several occasions. Step Four is the making of a searching and fearless moral inventory of one's life; taking time to reflect and write down times you know you've behaved badly towards self and others. The Fifth Step is where the rubber hits the road: "We admit to God, to ourselves, and to another human being the exact nature of our shortcomings." In this step the person who has made an inventory sits with a listener who simply hears the confession of all the "sins" one has made. It's a difficult step for many of us to endure.

Here's the amazing part of this moral inventory: As the observer/listener/confessor, most times I've listened to someone's Fifth Step and thought, sometimes said, "Is that it? Is that all? *That's* what you're still holding on to?" Because often, in someone's head, their transgressions are horrible, and their sins brand them as a deplorable or undesirable human being... yet we all have such acts and thoughts in our past. A good listener doesn't need to judge those acts and thoughts, only to hear them. As we express our transgressions and are heard by another, we're somehow transformed to realize we may not be the worst person on the planet after all. It's my belief that all of us live in a fear: "If they *really* knew me, they wouldn't like me." Learn to both like and forgive yourself!

Can You See Yourself Well?

Find reasons to want to get better; to stay alive, to thrive. If you can't find such reasons, chances are any challenge, including surgery, will be more difficult, with complications more likely to arise. Do you know the story of Viktor Frankl in *Man's Search for Meaning*?[8] A psychiatrist trained by Sigmund Freud and a Jew, Frankl was incarcerated in a concentration camp during World War II. As a student of the mind he decided to observe

8   V. Frankl (1984) *Man's Search for Meaning.* New York: Simon & Schuster.

the behavior of those around him as a purpose for keeping him alive. He noted that prisoners who had a reason to stay alive had a far better chance of surviving than those who seemed to have lost their purpose, reason and will. Whether a positive purpose like reuniting loved ones, or a negative one like getting revenge when their incarceration was finished…it didn't matter what sort of purpose was shown. Any strong feelings toward any purpose helped the prisoners stay alive.

What turns you on? *Why* do you want to get better? It may be as simple as the grandkids, or your partner, or your garden, or your pet, or your volunteer or paid work, or even the redecoration of the living room. It doesn't matter how trivial a purpose may seem to others; what makes you tick? Find it, honor it, nurture it and use it to talk yourself into wanting to heal quickly and completely so you can get back to joy, and you'll be more likely to do just that. And when you find people who support your purpose, you're well on your way to health, because you've found people who make the journey more fun.

I can't remember now where I read this, but one of the top psychologists years ago is reputed to have suggested that he could "cure" depression in nearly anyone…by giving the depressed person an assignment to help others! It makes sense that when you look at someone less fortunate and decide to assist them it will help to take your mind off your own problems. It may even make your problems seem very small indeed when you look around at how fortunate you are. That attitude of gratitude can guide us if we let it.

After my 1987 plane wreck and the surgery that fused my spine and installed steel rods to stabilize it, I decided I wanted to play the role of Don Quixote in "Man of La Mancha" before I gave up on life. I cast all the roles in my head from the members of a church choir I directed. I visualized the production in our church sanctuary. I used this image to motivate me to get better. It took over a year, but we had our production, I met my goal, and I strengthened my body, my connectedness and my purpose.

You are ultimately responsible for whether you get better or not. Others can help you, and many want to help you. But if you can't find the energy to get up and take the first steps, no amount of work from others can guarantee that you can get better. **It's *your* brain that's got to change; no one else can do it for you.**

Among the problems we might find in the head and neck: headaches, tumors, temporomandibular joint problems (TMJ), anxiety, panic disorders, insomnia, overall pain through the body, "fogginess" in the brain, strokes, mental illnesses, memory and dementia issues, shoulder problems, as well as sensory problems with vision, smell, hearing, taste and so on. When the brain is overwhelmed, the body must follow.

I often think of a turtle…when it feels safe, the head pulls out of the shell and the turtle moves through life. As soon as any danger shows itself, that turtle pulls the head, snap! Back into the body. In some ways, I think we've done that to ourselves, and science is starting to come around to this image, realizing that health in the neck and head can create health through the body. I believe if we could simply keep our head up, waist back, and allow the neck to be long and flexible, we'd have far fewer problems with this head center, because energy could reach it. Explore keeping a long and healthy neck with a "good head on your shoulders." What have you got to lose? In Chapter 6 on movement we'll focus on a few ways one can open and "oil" this neck to provide better energy to the head (see the exercises *A Good Head on Our Shoulders, Still the Shoulders, Arms: The Front Legs, Hanging from the Front Legs, An All Purpose Cue*).

Making the decision to be healthier and having the motivation to achieve this health is up to you. Are you ready? Are you interested? Do you want to "get ahead"? Or would you prefer to continue letting others decide what's appropriate health care for you, even to the point of letting go of your power, abdicating to "authorities" who see you more as a body, or a gall bladder, or a bad back, instead of a person who needs guidance and help on their journey?

We often suggest one turns to God for healing. This is an appropriate response. We also suggest "Ask for what you want (healing)." This too is appropriate. Sadly, too many of us turn to the doctor, and ask for someone to do for us instead of deciding to do for ourselves, with help from God and those around us. We'd prefer to "order from the menu" of health care, instead of changing our behaviors. Are you ready to rewire your brain for change, self-responsibility and true health? Easy to ask, difficult to choose.

The Heart: Healthy Circulation and Respiration Create a Healthy Flow

What good is your body if your heart's not in it?

For me, the heart is the **workhorse** of the body…the member who keeps us going. The beating of the heart moves the blood through the body's circulatory system, which both feeds and cleanses every cell. I believe it also engages the respiratory system which purifies the blood in the lungs and returns clean blood to the heart, enhancing the flow of lymphatic drainage through the body—our body's septic system. Think of the heart as the pump that moves nutrition through the body…if it's not healthy and happy, we're getting static, and dying—perhaps slowly, but dying nonetheless.

Just as we all realize the importance of the brain, the control panel of the body, we all know the heart's clear necessity. We talk about "broken hearts" and "having our heart in the right place." We write songs of love and heart yearning. But we forget what an amazing piece of machinery it really is, pumping blood through the body day and night for years on end. Heart health is critical. And we can't have a healthy heart if we won't remember to breathe.

It's such a simple, sad truth: We need to breathe better, more often and more deeply! For years I've witnessed clients get on my table, "relax" and begin a treatment. Usually I'll start our time together, especially on our first appointment, by asking to see a few good deep breaths. I'm often amazed at how little breath goes through most of us. Many people seem to totally hold their breath and resist filling the lungs; others seem to take quick and shallow breaths and think they're breathing. Most practitioners of yoga or tai chi understand that breath is critical. Breath is the ultimate fuel! Without air there is no life. Most of us seem to act as if there may not be enough oxygen in the atmosphere. Too many of us seem to believe that by breathing deeply, we're depriving self or the Universe of some energy…energy that might go more appropriately to someone or something else. Wrong!

Heart Rate Variability Indicates Health

With the breath comes heart health: Scientists are currently studying a measurement called *heart rate variability* (HRV).[1] HRV is an accurate indicator of health. When our nervous system functions well and we're socially engaged and able to find/face/feel and forget, our heart will beat at different rates as we breathe in (faster) or out (slower). A high HRV (meaning someone's heart can beat faster when inhaling or taxed, and really slow when relaxing, resting and exhaling) allows one to have less heart problems, diabetes, inflammations such as arthritis and fibromyalgia and mental/anxiety conditions. So clearly having a larger HRV number is a goal. HRV is the best predictor of health; the lower the HRV, the more likely we are to have illness and even die.

Now: Interestingly, we're beginning to see research suggesting the simplest way to enhance HRV is with structured breathing![2] It's been found that all of us have an optimal breath

---

1   HeartMath Institute (n.d.) Home page. Accessed on 13/05/2019 at www. heartmath.org/articles-of-the-heart/the-math-of-heartmath/heart-rate-variability.

2   M. De Couck *et al.* (2019) "How breathing can help you make better decisions." *International Journal of Psychophysiology 139*, 1–9.

rate…for most of us in the range of 4.5–7 breaths per minute. This means that if we'd simply sit or lie quietly for five or so minutes occasionally and focus on breathing in for roughly four seconds, out for five, and resting one second, we'd be altering our breath rate, our body's chemistry, and our heart rate health. And it's free!

My family doctor, Ralph, happens to also be my brother-in-law, and I feel blessed that when I have a need to discuss medical questions, I have a caring physician who listens, then offers information and advice. I've asked him to contribute to this book, and he'll appear in the next section. But he sees such importance in HRV that he asked to be quoted here as well:

> Basically, when we are sitting quietly, as we breathe in, our heart rate goes up, and as we breathe out, our rate goes down. HRV is the difference between these two heart rates. The greater our HRV, the better our overall health. A higher HRV is one of the best predicters of overall health. The lower one's HRV, the more likely the person is to die not only from heart disease, but any and all causes of death. This information is not new— the initial studies were done in the 1980s. We can increase our HRV by cardiovascular exercise and by slow and mindful breathing. It's been shown that end-stage heart disease patients waiting for a heart transplant can increase their HRV and improve their overall quality of life, by spending 20 minutes a day practicing slow mindfulness breathing. Increasing our HRV can dramatically strengthen our ability to self-regulate or self-modulate.

In addition to training our brain to have relaxing, positive thoughts about one's health instead of visualizing the worst case, can we learn to put slow and intentional breath into our systems? It makes sense we feel more balanced when we relax and allow joy and breath to flow through our body. Intentional breathing can enhance our HRV, reset our nervous network's "fight/flee/freeze" system and allow us to feel safer in the moment and healthier in our being. We're back to breath, relaxation and mindfulness. The more we can mindfully choose to activate our parasympathetic system and decide we're not really in danger, the more our nervous system can do its job. We'll catch our breath, our HRV will increase and we'll be healthier.

Consider the lymphatic and immune systems as also involved with our heart; the lymphatics trap and then flush the toxicities that have somehow been slowed and finally stopped from our body. The endocrine system releases chemicals into the body appropriately so we manage our daily activities with the needed doses of hormones. This system includes the adrenal glands which regulate that "fight or flee" aspect of movement. We become ill when we go static; without respiration and circulation, it's hard to create movement.

Feel the Fear

Spindler suggests in *Yoga Therapy for Fear* that we could all benefit from a simple walking/breathing awareness: She recommends a calming and enhancing of HRV with an aware walk, breathing in for four steps and breathing out for four steps as one walks. Can you envision how such a simple, yet profound exercise as a mindful walk will allow you to return to feelings of calm, enhance the breath rate and therefore the HRV, and bring you back to your "feel" state instead of your fight/flee/freeze position on the dial? Wise words!

Levine has demonstrated that much post-traumatic stress disorder (PTSD) can be alleviated with his reasonably simple (not easy!) technique of asking a client to revisit their traumatic place while paying attention to body sensations. As clients return to the trauma of their past, Levine asks "What's going on in your body? What do you notice now? Is anything changing?" When he or his practitioners work with such a client, they'll keep a sharp eye to make sure they're not overstimulating that client or pushing them back into the trauma too deeply; that's counter-productive. But if Levine can get the client to face the trauma while staying anchored in body sensations, often they as a team can finally resolve that old trauma's hold and return to the "feel" mode in the client's body. It's a talent we could all emulate; to stay in our bodies, examine our fears and dangers, and choose to process and self-regulate instead of hiding from, running from or fighting the danger.

Research projects also point to the fact that those of us who are socially engaged tend to be happier and live longer. Couples of long standing tend to be healthier and survive longer than single people or people in unhappy or unfulfilling couplings. And exclusive partnership seems less important to me; it's social connectedness that causes people to feel loved and needed, helping us stay happy and interested in being alive. Social connectedness can come from a happy primary partnership or a happy family life. But it may also come from a treasured pet, a treasured hobby, good friends, internet relationships, meaningful work or any number of connectors.

Many of us have heard of the five love languages…most of us demonstrate our love in one of these five ways, and usually perceive love coming most appropriately through one of these five languages as well. The five languages are acts of service, positive words, gifts, quality time or physical touch. If you as a person crave physical touch from a partner who believes words are the way to demonstrate love, the relationship can't be its fullest. When we learn to find another's style of receiving love and can use it instead of the language in which we're most proficient, we create a happier relationship. It serves us all to both know our personal love language that makes us feel secure and loved, and to understand that others may have a different language and we may want to learn to speak their language as well as training them to speak ours, if they're truly important to us.

For years I've suggested to clients that they might experiment with what I call "opening the heart hinge." It seems that between much of the work we do (computing, driving, craft work) and the feeling of emotional protection (early development of height or breasts, childhood emotional abuse, or feelings of unworthiness) many of us choose to collapse the area of our chest where our heart lives. Can you see how such a collapse could lead to extra tension in the heart area, and put further strain on the muscle? I often suggest someone learn to let their heart be the first center of the body to arrive in any situation. As you think of this idea, can you feel your body reacting by shortening its front face? The exercises *Bend, Twist, Flex, Twist and Turn, Side Flexion* and *Arms: The Front Legs* will help you with this idea of keeping an open heart hinge.

In addition to cardiovascular issues, congestive heart failure, atrial fibrillation, aneurisms and other heart issues, this closed heart hinge area can often lead to problems with the lungs and the breath as well as the head and neck *and* to shoulder and arm problems—if the hinge is closed, it suggests we've been collapsing our spine forward. Our control panel and our workhorse have gotten too close together! Whenever energy gets slowed, disease ensues.

So "if our heart's in it" and we have a healthy and happy heart, we enhance circulation, respiration, lymphatic flow, immune system and HRV, contributing to overall health and a decrease in many of the challenges we face in the body. What have you got to lose? Open your heart and let your body accept circulation…move stuck energy!

3

The Gut: Healthy Nutrition Provides a Healthy Fuel

Clean fuel makes a clean machine.

According to Ida Rolf in *Ida Rolf Talks about Rolfing and Physical Reality*,[1] near the turn of the nineteenth century into the twentieth, a French scientist named Claude Bernard was awarded the Légion d'Honneur and began his acceptance speech with the words "Gentlemen, a man is something built around a gut." It's an interesting concept to think that the mouth is one end, the anus is the other, and everything that comes into and out of the body needs to follow this gut path. I see the gut as the **processor/factory worker/server** of the body…that which deals with raw materials, creates a product, then disposes of it after the product has served its purpose…the original recycling center. When our gut becomes a dump it's in trouble and our body will be in trouble as well.

Some of us really want to succeed and achieve in life and accomplish grand goals; others simply want a good hamburger or the perfect ice cream and will drive across town to find it. Can you motivate yourself to put better fuel into your system? What sort of nutrition do you give your body? Do you eat healthy, organic, and eat to live? Or do you make a production

---

1   R. Feitis (1978) *Ida Rolf Talks about Rolfing and Physical Reality.* New York: Harper and Row.

of food intake and live to eat? Do you monitor your diet, or grab fast foods with little nutrition in them? Choose wisely; one is killing you and one is keeping you healthy. Remember earlier we challenged ourselves to make any movement and take tiny steps forward. Can you see how this hunting/gathering for the correct fuel for your body can be one of the first steps you can take to make yourself healthy?

Let's begin thinking about the nutrition we provide our bodies by visiting the basic element we're all most comprised of, in our bodies—water. One could see water as the lubricant and the fuel of our machinery, that which helps our body to run smoothly. We're also aware that without water we'd not be on the planet; in fact, water can be seen as the ground substance of our planet. Not only could we not survive; all creatures, plant and animal, depend on water as well. Our bodies and our planet are about 70–80 percent water; thus without water we'd be reduced to nearly nothing. Second, try living without food, shelter, social contact and water; water (and air) will quickly demand our attention! Movement and appropriate fuel can change a static body into a *fluid* one. The kidneys, also located in the gut center, are associated with this water element, and with good reason: The kidneys need water flow to filter all that comes into and goes out of the body. When water doesn't move, through us or through our world, the static and stagnant nature of us is enhanced. We become more toxic, more poisoned, all the way to the bones. The healthier and more hydrated we are and the cleaner the fuel we install in our systems, the happier our bodies will be, especially if we'll simply get up and move a bit as well.

The liver is also in the stomach cavity/lumbar plexus segment of the body, as are pancreas and spleen. All these organs function in ways that either store and process toxicities, regulate chemicals or in some way act as a filter to purify body elements so we can function appropriately. All are important workers in the abdomen's factory. This gut area is so important to overall health!

Poor eating habits contribute to so many issues: digestive and eliminative issues, certainly, but ulcers, gall bladder problems, liver issues, splenic and pancreatic issues, diabetes, kidney infections and other problem. The list is incomplete because it could be argued every problem in the body may be served by putting better fuel in the system!

You Are What You Drink

Most of us don't drink enough water; I'd argue most of us don't take in as much as our body would like. Think of it less as the fuel and more as the oil for the body. If you run your machinery without oil, it will wear out much sooner. Coffee, tea, sodas, alcohol and fruit juices aren't water, though they have elements of water in them. If you're going to use any of them as a substitute, I suppose green tea comes closest to water…and one could water down fruit juices. There is actually no substitute for good old water.

A word about bottled waters: We're beginning to find that many "healthy" waters actually contain toxicities…some "spring" water seems to be bottled right from the tap! Beyond this, water can react with the plastic in its bottle and become toxic to us as a result. If you insist on using bottled waters, consider whether your brand is truly pure water, and don't leave bottles in storage for long periods of time, especially in warm or sunny environments!

We all realize that without water, air and fuel we couldn't survive. Yet most of us breathe shallowly if at all, hardly drink water (some who "just don't like the taste of it") and eat foods that have had most of the life force processed out of them. Can you, either in preventative mode or as preparation for your surgery, add to your intake of pure water? We've all heard the formula: Your body weight in pounds divided by two is equal to the number of ounces of water you should be drinking daily. Warning: I believe you can also drink too much water. I think you can overhydrate and leach important minerals from your system by this overhydrating. But if constipation is, has been, or becomes an issue, visit your water intake.

If water sounds boring, flavor it with cranberry concentrate from the health food store or a bit of lemon juice…no sugar, only cranberry or lemon. You could even add a touch of carbonated water such as club soda for that "fizz." A small dose in a large glass or sipper of ice water can last for hours but delivers constant vitamin C and a gentle antibiotic effect in addition to the body's lubrication. Cranberry concentrate was one of the few necessary items in my hospital kit when I had both surgeries recently.

Your Water Is Also How You Think!

I'm reminded of a fascinating photo book called *The Messages from Water* by Masuro Emoto.[2] Scientist Emoto began viewing various samples of water through a microscope and was stunned by the results. The photos in his book show amazing changes in the organization of water when emotions come into play.

Specifically, water is susceptible to our thoughts and feelings, and to its physical and emotional environment! Water that receives or is surrounded by "good energy" or positive emotional messages exhibits a more crystalline, organized structure, while water that is in some way made to feel a slowed-down energy becomes denser, more chaotic and uglier. Some of Emoto's simple experiments involved verbally or emotionally berating a water sample, cursing, sending bad energy towards that sample; then watching such water become more chaotic in structure. On the other hand, water that was loved, praised, given good energy instead of anger, seemed to form more crystalline and beautiful structures.

Water that is "fed" with Mozart's music playing displays beauty and crystallinity; water bombarded with heavy metal "music" can't seem to find any sort of structure whatsoever.

---

2   M. Emoto (2000) *The Messages from Water.* Tokyo: Hado.

What thoughts are we putting into the water in our bodymindcore system? Remember, according to science, we're at least 80 percent water in our bodies. How are we treating this water? What do we say to it/us? Are we feeding ourselves positive emotions and thoughts in addition to positive foods and drinks?

You Are What You Eat, Too

What's your relationship to food? Do you enjoy healthy foods, or do you enjoy everything you see? Can you moderate your intake, or do you just love the tastes so much that you can't stop? Can you still eat a large pizza all by yourself? Do you need a little sugar or a little coffee to get you going? Do you realize how much your body suffers from junk food and sodas instead of fruit smoothies and vegetables? Can you focus on several small meals a day instead of one or two huge meals? Diet is critical at any stage, and the more attention we pay to a healthy diet the more rewards we're likely to find.

We realize more and more both how foods are more poisonous than they were 50 years ago, but also how few foods are truly real and healthy food at all. These days we live on "food products." Recently someone suggested to me that when visiting a grocery store I could totally ignore the inner aisles and visit only the periphery. I was amazed to realize that nearly everything with any real food value and vitality was on the outer edges of the store: The produce department, the dairy, meats, baked goods and health foods usually are all on the outer edges (some dairy, yogurt and eggs now live in a center aisle near the checkouts). Common sense has always told us that the less like the original food a product has become, probably the less total food value it possesses.

By no means do I consider myself a nutritionist, and by no means can I advise all of us on the best diet for every individual! I can, however, suggest that the freshest, least processed food we ingest in moderate amounts, chances are the healthier and happier we'll be. As we look at the food value of most grocery items, let's simply consider which contain water and which are dried, processed and have the water drained away, taking their nourishment in too many cases. Produce, dairy, meats— all continue to store water, while chips, crackers and other snack foods lack water, and *vitality*. Water is one of the vital essences; energy being another. While we can't exactly define and quantify energy, we can absolutely work on enhancing our water intake.

Here's an interesting thought: Begin to truly look at your foods as either medicine or poison. Chances are the purest unflavored water and the freshest and least processed foods are your medicine and the foods and drinks least recognizable from their original form are poisonous. None of us is created exactly the same, having the same bacteria in our digestive system, and none of us are built with the same chemistry as everyone else on the planet. Therefore, each of us will have a diet that works best for us...can we look for it? Some thrive on protein, especially meat. Others believe in fruitarian or vegetarian or vegan diets. What works for you, that seems healthy as well?

Which seems to be more healing: apple juice with sugar, or an apple? A grilled or sautéed filet of fish, or fish sticks? A chicken breast or chicken nuggets? Milk or ice cream? Whole grain flour or refined and processed flour or breads? How far from its original state is this food?

> Begin to truly look at your foods as either medicine or poison. Chances are the purest unflavored water and the freshest and least processed foods are your medicine and the foods and drinks least recognizable from their original form are poisonous.

There are volumes of books written to tell us how to eat the healthiest foods; for our blood type, to save our heart, to lose (or gain) weight, to stimulate ketosis, to balance our energies and so on, and so on. Everybody has a take on what feeds our bodymindcores most efficiently and healthily. I have my take as well, based on what I've already said: Choose fresh, choose that which looks like it looked when it was harvested. Choose the liveliest foods you can find, and then choose to eat less of them than you really want to eat! And that can be the toughest part for many of us.

Table 3.1 Are *your* foods medicine, poison, or a little bit of both? Where do *you* fit on this chart?

MEDICINES	NEUTRAL	POISONS
Fresh coldwater fish	Frozen fish	Too much meat, especially beef. Store-roasted chicken
Organ meats, bone broth	Chicken, turkey	'Luncheon' meat/cold cuts
Organic chicken/ turkey	Lamb, pork	
Most fresh fruits and vegetables	Leafy greens, raw	Vegetable chips/ products
"Roots and fruits" (organic, lightly cooked is best)		
Almond/soy/coconut/ hemp "milks"	Fermented milk products	Soft cheeses, milk
Kefir	Hard cheeses	Ice cream
Most nuts and seeds	Organic nut butters	Grocery nut butters
Water, green tea	Fruit and vegetable juices	Sodas, alcohol
Lemon and cranberry concentrate	Coffee and tea (no sugar)	Energy drinks
Butter, coconut oil (best for cooking)	Olive oil, extra virgin	Margarine
Olive oil raw		Trans fats/ polyunsaturated oils
Yogurt without fruit	Yogurt sugared with fruit	Frozen yogurt

cont.

MEDICINES	NEUTRAL	POISONS
Avocados	Dark chocolate small amounts	Milk chocolate, candy
Honey in small amounts, Manuca is best	Date sugar, stevia	Cane and beet sugars
	Agave in small amounts	Corn syrup
		Artificial sweeteners
Quinoa	Rice, whole grains	Processed white flour
Cauliflower as a grain		
Some current dieticians suggest that in hunter-gatherer style, we do best eating 30 percent animal based protein (organic clearly best), 20 percent carbohydrates including very little grains with more veggies and fruit with few sugars, and 50 percent fats and oils, though not polyunsaturated or trans-fats. Again, you are your own best authority: What makes you feel well?		

As you look at this chart, do you see how many of the medicinal foods are both fresher, more alive, and have more water in them? Again, common sense suggests that live foods enhance your water intake, while poisoned and processed foods demand even more water intake if they're to be diluted and digested. We know and understand the need for water; will we honor it?

And we're beginning to finally understand the gut and the amazing biomes we have in it; the plethora of bacteria fulfilling so many functions! Sometimes nasty bacteria rears its ugly head: *E. coli*, for example. Our body will deal with such an intruder; but think how easy life would be if we kept healthy bacteria in our gut so it could deal more quickly and easily with those outliers that try to do damage. An interesting book by Giulia Enders is called *Gut: The Inside Story of Our Body's Most Under-Rated Organ*.[3] This fine book encourages us to really understand the intricacies of our digestive and eliminative system. Among other fascinating information, she offers new

---

3   G. Enders (2015) *Gut: The Inside Story of Our Body's Most Under-Rated Organ.* Vancouver/Berkeley, CA: Greystone Books.

research showing that stress also affects digestion, elimination and health of gut flora! We know we should eat better foods, and more alive foods *as we stay relaxed*. Will we?

In *Gut* we learn that bacteria make up most of the population in our gut…and each of us has, like a fingerprint, our personal inventory of bacteria in the gut (unlike a fingerprint, however, that inventory can constantly change). In the last few years we've even come to realize that certain bacteria in our gut probably have influence on the body's overall metabolism, thus, possibly/probably, even our weight. Certain bacteria seem to be more common in overweight people, while others are missing. And if certain metabolism problems such as obesity and diabetes indicate higher levels of infection markers in blood, we're beginning to trace those problems to specific bacteria which are missing or rampant in individuals. As mild-grade infections in the gut also cause weight gain (along with other factors such as hormone imbalances, too much estrogen, lack of vitamin D and too much gluten-rich food), it's possible people with weight issues simply need a bacteria transplant! If we could change that gut fingerprint, would more people be able to lose, or gain, weight?

Another fascinating idea from *Gut*: it's been hypothesized since 2013 that gut bacteria may be the cause for some out-of-control appetites on our part. While we all love to protest "It's not my fault!" and many of us know we seem to lack will power when it comes to food intake, it's possible it's actually *not* your appetite that's out of control! It may be your bacteria or parasites are the hungry ones, not you.

Recent studies also suggest we're healthier when we limit the amount of time in the day when we intake our food and drink. Optimally, if we eat from morning till late afternoon, in perhaps an eight- to ten-hour shift, we seem to be healthier and able to keep weight off more easily. Think about your current situation: Like many of us, do you have your morning coffee with perhaps a pastry at 7 am, then continue eating until 9 or 10 in the evening, ending with that last glass of wine just before bed? Some authorities even suggest a type of fast where one only eats between the hours of noon and 5 pm. It's very difficult to live on this planet and follow that type of structure! Yet a shorter window of time to ingest, digest and a longer window to rest seems helpful. Give your gut's factory workers occasional time off! Play with the idea that perhaps the bowl of ice cream might be healthier just after an early dinner rather than just before bed.

The Bowels

Bowel movements! Probably the older one gets, the more important this topic becomes...prune juice, psyllium, Dieter's Tea, probiotics, Dulcolax, Miralax, more water, and so on, and so on...common sense tells us if waste products aren't leaving, we'll develop physical issues from the inner toxins. Keeping a relaxed attitude, a healthy diet and a calmed nervous system can contribute to regular and healthy bowel movements. Have you ever noticed how most young children have large, soft yet firm stools, while older people who have been eating and living incorrectly for too long, often have small, tight, hard stools? We've lost the way.

An interesting research project from Japan again reaffirms common sense. Realize that in many countries, people squat to have their bowel movements instead of sitting on a toilet. In those countries, we see far fewer back and bowel problems than we see in "civilized" countries. Japanese researchers have realized that squatting does make a clearer, straighter open channel for feces to exit the body, and that many diseases or conditions such as hemorrhoids, diverticulitis and even constipation are nearly unknown in countries where people squat to evacuate their bowels.[4]

On the market in the USA today, one can find a product called "Squatty Potty." Its purpose is to duplicate that squatting

4   R. Sakakibara *et al.* (2010) "Influence of body position on defecation in humans." *LUTS* 2, 1, 16–21.

posture during bowel movements. It's simply a small stool in a U-shaped curve that wraps around the base of your toilet, then slides forward so you can put your feet on the stool and enhance the channel in your colon to facilitate easier bowel movements. Again, common sense.

If we go back to the idea that movement helps our body, no matter what our issue, can you see how a bit of movement in the middle of the body could help with digestion and elimination? I'd recommend visiting twisting, lateral flexion and forward and back movements as great ways to help keep the extra pounds and to keep foods moving through you. See *Bend, Twist, Flex, Twist and Turn, Side Flexion, Opening the Sacroiliac Junctions* and *Animal Walks* for ideas that assist the gut in staying open and energized.

What's Your Fuel?

We all know we could and should be eating healthier diets, even as we rationalize: "I don't have energy after a long day at work to prepare something healthy and nutritious." "I have so little free time that I just grab a burger or donut and a cup of coffee, and that's how I fuel myself for that long day." "Decent, and especially organic foods, are just so expensive!" "I just don't seem to be able to control my appetite; I'll eat even when I'm full simply because I'm enjoying the tastes so much!" All our rationalizations may be true, but we all know that if we eat moderately, sparingly, and eat to live instead of living to eat, fueling our system with fresher and fewer processed foods in moderate amounts, we'll be far healthier. If you're interested in remaining healthy, why not explore cleaner and more moderate eating for at least a week or two and see if you feel differently?

Let's don't even get me started on both sugar and the "replacements" that have been invented. In the first place, I think we all could admit we use too much sugar, especially corn syrup, which is now an ingredient in far too many "foods," and very possibly contributing to the obesity epidemic prevalent in most "civilized" countries. Nearly every food product we buy lists sugar as an ingredient and often a main one, though it may be disguised under one of perhaps 30 different names. The best way to cut back on sugar is both to learn what names you'll find it listed under in ingredients, and to cook for yourself with fresh natural ingredients without added sugar. Even pasta, spaghetti sauce, salad dressings and catsup are filled with sugar! Clearly, sugar contributes to inflammation and feeds bacteria. Is this really what you want in your system when you're deciding to be more health conscious?

And the artificial sweeteners that are still being pushed on us are potentially even worse. Internet searches will highlight links between sweeteners and several conditions including cancer, ADHD, weight gain or inability to lose weight, diabetes, migraines, fibromyalgia and food allergies. Limiting sugar intake and staying off artificial substances of any kind continue to be sensible steps when preparing to enter and stay in hospital during and after surgery. If you can't stop the habit, at least try to cut back on your intake and up your water intake!

It's documented that for years the sugar industry has been aware of the health risks of high sugar intake. Their solution was to create an ad campaign nothing short of genius: They began blaming health problems on too much fat in the diet and hired researchers who could find results that supported this claim. Consequently, most of us stayed with our sugar enjoyment but avoided even the healthy fats. Now we're realizing that "good" fats are necessary to our health, after years of believing they were the major culprit.

Whatever you put into your body—the liquids, the solids, the chemicals, the medications and the junk food, or even the thoughts and affirmations you're introducing into your brain as we talked about earlier—all are critical to health. Just as we can't be healthy if we won't honor our thoughts and prayers and keep them in a nutritious realm instead of a negative one, we can't live a healthy life eating and drinking only that which is bad for us.

4

The Groin: Healthy Regeneration Invites a Healthy Future

When in danger, we tuck our tails and tighten our pelvic floors.

I continue to believe one of my primary sources of inspiration, previously mentioned author and researcher Stephen Porges, has hit on a critical issue when he suggests, referring to mental and physical health: "the pivotal point is, can we get people to feel safe?" If we can't feel and experience rest and relaxation, how do we stay well? If we don't believe our shelter is safe and secure, what kind of world do we inhabit?

How can we grow if we can't feel safe, rested and relaxed? How do we branch out if we're afraid to stretch towards sunlight and open space? How do we get rooted if we can't allow ourselves to dig in, absorb that which is around us as nutrition and carry on with living? As we unwind the tension that lives deep in our core, at the very "root" of our being, in our survival chakra area of the groin, we find a relaxed and balanced state that allows us to run our bodymindcores more efficiently.

I find the body systems most related to this groin element are the reproductive and eliminative systems of the body…that which not only allows our "tight ass" condition to release and resolve, but which also insures the survival of our species.

Rebooting Your Mental Computer

What sort of thoughts are you feeding your bodymindcore? Do they relax you and make you feel safe, or do they create stress? Too many of us continue to beat ourselves up: "I'm not good enough. I don't do enough. Nobody likes me. What's the use? It's a cold cruel world." Do you affirm your worth and your joy in the world, or do you continue to sit unhappily in your chair and endure life as it goes by? How safe and contented do you feel in your world?

Visualize. Affirm. Claim the joy you want in your life. For years, three of my favorite affirmations have been these:

- Every day in every way I'm giving better and better.

- I am satisfied with my progress and my process.

- I am worthy of self-respect.

The first of these is based on an affirmation attributed to Emile Coué. A psychotherapist and student of human nature over one hundred years ago, he coined the phrase "optimistic autosuggestion" and believed the use of such self-affirming words could enhance physical and mental health. His words and intent were a bit different than my affirmation above, as he suggested, "Every day in every way I'm *getting* better and better." While this is a fantastic affirmation to use, personally I've enjoyed exchanging that word "getting" for the word "giving." It seems to me that if we could all focus on and contribute to the good around us and fixate less on fear inside, we'd be happier. I've been using this affirmation for years.

The second concept…satisfaction. So important! Years ago, our clinic group held weekly meetings for improvement of selves and our clinic. One day we discussed the "perfect affirmation." One colleague suggested "I am satisfied." I stated this idea didn't work for me because if some one-celled being had called itself satisfied millions of years ago, we wouldn't have striven and evolved into who and what we are today. He then amended: "How about, I'm satisfied with my progress?" I thought that was about perfect, and still use it often. A client, on hearing this phrase, suggested adding "…and my process" to the affirmation. I really like this! "I'm satisfied with my progress and my process." Neither affirmation suggests I've arrived at that final and perfect destination; only that I give myself credit for the journey I've made thus far.

And last: "I am worthy of self-respect." I believe this one is perhaps the most powerful of the affirmations I've found. Most of us still wrestle with thoughts of not being good enough. If we can't respect ourselves, warts and all, why should we expect others to respect us? Without being too proud, or a bully, or a braggart, we can develop an attitude that affirms "I am enough." I affirm daily, for about 500 steps of 2500 around my house— each 100 steps emphasizes a different word—I am worthy of self-respect. I **am** worthy of self-respect. I am **worthy** of self-respect. Another 500 steps are devoted to you—**You** are worthy…Powerful words! Another 1000 steps are devoted to "Every day in every way I'm **giving** better and better" and "Every day in every way I'm **getting** better and better". Remember: *The Message of Water* suggests that how we think and feel about ourselves creates the being we become.

> What sort of thoughts are you feeding your body-mindcore? Do they relax you and make you feel safe, or do they create stress? Too many of us continue to beat ourselves up: "I'm not good enough. I don't do enough." I've basically decided that as I'm doing the best job I know how to do in most situations, *even with some small misfires or mistakes, I'm good enough,* and I deserve to continue moving forward into an even better world.

Can you say any of these affirmations aloud and mean it, and believe it? This can be extremely difficult for most of us, but if you can allow yourself to look in a mirror, make eye contact, and use any of these three sentences while you pay attention to your body, I think you'll have an eye-opening experience.

It's interesting to just monitor your thoughts and your body's response when you experiment with positive self-talk. Too many of us only use negative talk when dealing with our shortcomings, fears and shame instead of finding and focusing on the good parts of us.

Shame: The Root Fear?

Many of us have a hard time accepting any of my three affirmations above. I agree with author/lecturer Louise Hay, who suggests that at the root of most illness is a significant lack of self-esteem.[1] I've struggled with that self-esteem demon but, at this point in my life, partly through the above affirmations, I've basically decided that as I'm doing the best job I know how to do in most situations, *even with some small misfires or mistakes, I'm good enough*, and I deserve to continue moving forward into an even better world.

When one can believe they're good enough and doing enough, a great pressure is relieved. It's easier to move into the future more enthusiastically and positively. That's personal safety. Explore affirmations! They can work at any step of any difficult process: prevention, preparation or recovery. Do your mental work before, after and during interchanges with others...know yourself, what you need from your world and what you believe will happen. Frame it, visualize it, expect it and see it. Wag your tail and ungird your loins! Relax.

Now, take these ideas into the sexual realm of the body; realize too many of us see sexual feelings or activity as "shameful," and indeed, it seems many of us still try to hide from or ignore both our sexual apparatus and the feelings that arise from that area. Can we look at ourselves, honestly, truthfully, and decide that in every realm of our life and bodymindcore, including the sexual realm, we can be satisfied? We are enough? Every day in every way we're giving better and better? We're

---

1   L. Hay (1984) *You Can Heal Your Life*. Carlsbad, CA: Hay House.

worthy of self-respect? Can we let go of the shame we seem to hold when we think about, feel or discuss our sexual energy? Can we learn to celebrate our sexual aliveness?

Conditions which might occur when we have feelings of sexual shaming: overweight, underweight, difficult menstrual cycles, sexual dysfunction, migraine headaches, difficulty in conceiving and delivering, cystitis, fibroid tumors, ovarian or prostrate problems, incontinence or diarrhea, low back and tailbone pain or any other problems which seem to center around the groin area. Can you see how a slowdown of energy, caused by the feelings of shame too many of us have assigned to our sexual nature, could cause such difficulties? Can you allow your sexual energy to flow through your groin, and through you?

It's my theory that most of us are stuck in this groin energy; thus, energy can't rise further, into the gut, heart and head. By simply focusing on bringing breath, energy and awareness into the groin, then asking that energy to rise further into the gut and hopefully higher, we can allow ourselves to be open to an energetic flow throughout the body. I'll often lie on my back, put my hands on my stomach, and focus on bringing energy through the groin and towards the gut. On some days I can literally feel the movement beyond the gut, into the heart and occasionally into the head area. I consider this type of breath to be another reset of the vagus mechanism…simply finding energy all the way through the being seems to give the entire bodymindcore a good, deep exhale!

Exercises that can most help to keep open the groin center (as well as the low back and the legs) are *Down Stairs, Big Toe Pushups, Opening the Sacroiliac Junctions, Underthings: Hamstrings and Adductors, Hamstrings Alone* and *An Easier Hamstring Stretch*. As most of us live in shame in our groin area, these stretches that invite us to open, explore, find/face/feel and forget the shame can make huge changes in our bodymindcore, if we can be open to change.

One more idea fits in this concept of affirming that indeed we are what we think we are, especially for those oriented to the

Bible: In that book, when Moses meets God (Exodus 3:14) he asks His name. God responds, "My name is I AM." First, this simply suggests to me that God doesn't get mired in the past or the future, but in the precious present. Second, if indeed among the Ten Commandments we see a commandment to not take the name of the Lord in vain, it follows that we should be careful how we use God's name in a statement beginning with "I am." If we say "I am sick, I am tired, I am poor…" aren't we taking the name of I AM in vain? But if we can retrain ourselves to say, and think, "I am healthy, I am energized, I am wealthy…" aren't we creating a certain amount of health just by obeying the Commandment?

5

The Extremities: Healthy Motivation Insures a Healthy Ability

If one can't or won't find a reason to move, one won't get very far.

For many of us, the hardest part of any path to healing involves us first deciding to get up and move…to take steps towards that which we want. Why? Why is it so difficult to get motivated? Pete Egoscue in his book *Pain Free* suggests we all suffer from "motion starvation" and I believe he's right.[1] Why is it so hard to get up off the couch and make things happen? Why is it so much easier to read, or watch the TV, or talk or text on the phone or play with the iPad? Why have we turned so static, so unmoving, so like a block of metal? Some of us seem to be most comfortable sitting at home and crying. Why? Why do we grieve and fear instead of finding that which keeps us alive and moving?

Some researchers, Daniel Wolpert among them,[2] now suggest that, based on their studies of other creatures, it's

---

1   P. Egoscue with R. Gittines (2000) *Pain Free: A Revolutionary Method for Stopping Chronic Pain*. New York: Random House.

2   D. Wolpert (2011) *The Real Reason for Brains*. TED talk. Accessed on 13/05/2019 at www.ted.com/talks/daniel_wolpert_the_real_reason_for_brains.

possible we primarily have a brain so we'll be able to move! Sadly, for too many of us, our brain is so often shouting warning messages to us that we can't focus on the simple activities of movement. If we could disengage the mechanisms we've built on top of this simple brain activity, would we be healthy more of the time?

Other researchers such as Bud Craig theorize that human self-awareness originates in that part of the brain called the *insular cortex*.[3] As this area receives feedback from the entire body and processes feelings, Craig likewise suggests the purpose of the brain is foremost to create movement, and the aim of that movement is to change the status quo and accomplish a meaningful task. Our brain is created to help us move, and our extremities can't move if our brain (and heart, gut and groin) won't let them.

Many of us would rather stay in a static, stuck place instead of looking at our feelings that make us want to shrink into self when we're afraid of meeting the world. We'd prefer ending life instead of moving into it, tightening our core being for survival's sake instead of eagerly facing the world with open arms and limber legs. Movement is critical to health! It's critical to the connective tissue or fascial network—the system that wraps the muscles, provides structure and form not only around muscles, but also through them, as well as encasing and giving form to organs and to every part of the body. Ida Rolf called fascia "the organ of support" and I think this is a fair name. When we have structure, we can be healthy; when our structure declines, we decline as well.

Textbooks today still don't identify the connective tissue network as a traditional system of its own. While one could lump it in with the muscular and skeletal systems, in that all three provide support and structure, I think this fascial system deserves a spot of its own. First, like the grain in the wood

---

3   B. Craig (2015) *How Do You Feel?* Accessed on 13/05/2019 at brainsciencepodcast.com/bsp/121-craig.

of a tree, the fascia is continuous through the body. Second, it provides structure and support, but also communication between various body parts, and even between cells. We're studying fascia more diligently and beginning to learn fascinating nuggets about it. Begin to think of fascia as an important system that's finally beginning to get its due respect. Realize that when we find and honor our fascia, we create more health in our bodymindcores. Begin to see the arms and legs, the hands and feet, as extensions of that bodymindcore, and see that we can use them to accomplish great things, if we'll just move them! Remembering the old song about hipbone being connected to knee bone, and so on, one can truly see how anything that happens in the sleeve or extremities of the body must be initiating from somewhere deeper in the system. As a bodyworker, I rarely look at shoulder/arm/elbow/hand problems without thinking most specifically first of the shoulder and cervical or neck structure. I used to ask myself if the neck problem was coming from the shoulder, or the shoulder problem initiated in the neck…my answer became "yes."

Motivation to MOVE

My real introduction to the importance of movement came years ago when I visited a 93-year-old cousin in her nursing home residence. She could no longer get out of her chair, so, daily, attendants came to lift her from her chair, drape her onto her walker or Zimmer frame, and make her walk the length of the hall so they could chart her activity. The facility was called a Rehabilitation Center; yet I never saw anything that looked to me like rehabilitation. I always wondered: "Why don't they teach her how to develop strength in her arms so she can lift herself out of the chair and move forward under her own power?" It seemed to me then, and now, that the medical establishment often has different goals than I'd want to have in terms of helping people return to function.

I wondered if anyone ever suggested she simply put her hands on the arms of the chair and explore lifting herself out of it. I wouldn't expect her to be able to do so, but I thought that with a bit of patience and work she could lift herself again and at the least restore a bit of arm strength that would serve her in other activities. Even if she only became less heavy to lift, movement and exercise could only have a good effect. My father-in-law proves this point to me, as he can still live on his own at 95 because he continues to push himself to get out of his chair. These two elders got me exploring the pieces of furniture and structural features in my own home and office.

I began with a simple canvas deck chair and found that, in addition to that wonderful tilting back that allows the spine and neck to extend backwards, the hands and arms could be used for lifting my upper body off the chair arms. One can also sit in a deck chair, put both hands on one arm, and twist the upper body to first one side, then turn everything to the other side, with breath at every stage of the movement. Anchor both hands on one arm and twist as far as possible in that direction; then reverse. How hard is that? And why don't we try to do so a bit more often, in any seated situation?

The more I've thought about my experience with the cousin, and the more challenges I've experienced with slowed energy in my own body, the more I've come to realize **I need to move more slowly, deliberately, and with awareness and intention** if I'm to truly feel and honor my body as it moves through space. I've found that when I slow down my walk, for example, and pay attention to the way my left or right foot contacts the ground, I can begin to realize I'm withholding a bit of foot bed from the ground. I can feel that tightened strain translating up into my leg muscles and even into my back. I often remember that Ida Rolf, founder of the work I first studied, suggested maturity is the ability to discern finer distinctions (class notes from Peter Melchior, faculty member at the Rolf Institute). I think I'm maturing as a body! To that end, I'll offer a few of the ways I choose to see everything around me as exercise equipment. We don't need fancy equipment to help us move!

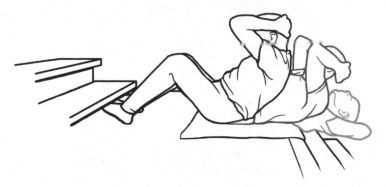

Using stairs as exercise equipment in a new way.

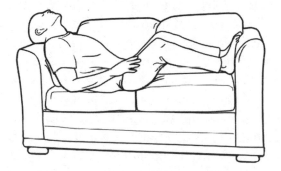

Exploring a divan arm as your bolster to open the heart hinge.

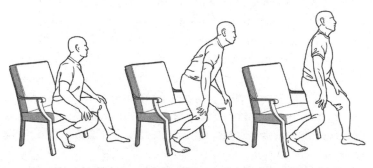

Developing arm strength by lifting in/out/in/out of the chair.

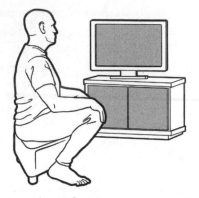

*Even watching television, you can practice
enhancing posture and movement.*

I've found that one of three things must happen to keep me moving: First, I decide I've got to get motivated and begin moving myself, walking, stretching, swimming daily and not letting myself "off the hook" just because I got up late, or it's too rainy, or any other excuse I can find. The second technique that often works for me, and might work for you, involves making a commitment, contract or promise to myself or someone I trust that some sincere and regular movement will happen, then figuring out how to keep that promise. One final way to insure one moves is to spend money! When I choose to invest in a month's worth of yoga classes, I'm more inclined to show up and work through the series, as I've paid for it. When I buy a service of bodywork I've invested both time and money energy, and I'm more likely to remember my exercises and homework. I invite you to decide which of these people you are: the self-motivator who can be faithful to the movements you know you need to make, the person who needs a friend/coach/cheerleader to whom they must report success or failure or the person who needs the motivation of paying someone to make sure you "get your money's worth." All can be effective—which could work for you?

I've offered the theory that we're so static because we can't seem to get motivated…not just the motivation of motion, but the motivation of doing things because we enjoy doing and feel like we contribute by doing them. Perhaps we might call this condition "motivation starvation" as well as motion starvation. Motivation is too lacking in too many of us. We jangle ourselves up and out of bed, struggling to motivate. We go to work, perhaps in a place we don't enjoy, or we stay at home in a situation where we see few people all day, and don't make real connections with others. It's been years since we needed to be hunters and gatherers and we've forgotten that there's a certain joy in getting up, getting out and taking on the world to see what it can bring us.

> I've offered the theory that we're so static because we can't seem to get motivated...not just the motivation of motion, but the motivation of doing things because we enjoy doing and feel like we contribute by doing them.

So, can you find a reason for moving? Are you ready to make the effort to get out of your chair and do an exercise or take a few steps? Are you ready to lose weight, or find a new job, or make new friends? Find something to motivate you—not too far-away a goal, hopefully achievable, and your body will decide to move more frequently and with enthusiasm it may currently lack. Be it a new grandchild, a renewal with your partner, a shift in attitude at your job or church, accepting aging gracefully, reaching retirement or any other motivator—find something to excite you and get those arms, legs and body moving, getting into the world or the parts you enjoy.

Awareness is such an important word! Yet many of us, in our automatic pilot mode, do what we can to avoid the sensations of our body. We crave positive sensation but hide from feeling what seems like "negative" feedback. Sorting through that negativity might lead us to the positive place, yet we're afraid to go looking. If we can't explore the negative, we can never truly move through it, into the positive movement sensations. And since we can't open the core we can't open the extremities.

Soon we'll offer stretches to help open and move arms and legs. Meanwhile, begin to stay aware of your awareness, or visit your lack of it, and consider moving more.

Every good deep tissue massage therapy textbook tells us that the deeper you want to go in a body or a system, the slower you go. This is true for movement *awareness* as well. Several schools of movement therapy use a simple technique: Practitioners ask a client to slow their movements and become more aware of each piece of activity, as well as their relation to space during movement. After the client explores and practices such a movement, the practitioner suggests "Now, do that twice as slowly." After a few more tries, the practitioner repeats the same suggestion. Getting clients to slow their actions and pay attention to smaller and smaller details can yield impressive realizations for that attentive client, and for any person who wants to gain health and stay healthy.

Sitting: Our Worst and Most Common Posture

Let's think specifically about sitting for a moment. Ida Rolf suggested sitting was the most difficult posture to achieve; standing was easier, and the simplest posture to maintain was lying down. Common sense, right? When you consider that it's relatively easy to have your body make a straight line while lying down, and a bit more challenging when standing (stop slumping!), you can see how, when sitting, you've put several kinks into that deep line before you even get on task.

We'll begin with this posture too many of us maintain too much of the time. It's hard to think of movement when one's body is anchored in one's bottom too often. But with a bit of thought and practice, even sitting can become a bit less detrimental to us all. Attention to the way we sit can make a big difference to both our posture and the way we feel. And as so many of us sit so much of the day, it pays to think about our personal seated posture: Which parts of you connect to the chair? Where do you "close off" the front of your body as you sit? What does lifting your head and shoulders upback and ceilingward feel like it does to your body?

And to get out of a chair, whether using arms or not, why not put one foot slightly behind the other, then use the back foot and leg to push yourself up and out of the chair instead of nolting the arms and back to take so much of the work? (See illustration on page 73.) Sadly, so many of our couches and chairs are very low, making it nearly impossible to get one leg behind the other and lift from the legs…but a bit of attention to using the legs to lift can make such a difference. Simply shifting the body sideways a bit, then lifting/pushing with that back leg, one can rise more easily.

In the last few years a study in Brazil found that older adults who needed to use hands and knees to rise to vertical from a cross-legged position on the floor lived fewer years than similarly aged people who could get up easily without using arms and knees. It makes sense…and recalls once again that old saying, "Use it or lose it."

This chapter on why movement is critical is shorter because we've talked about movement through the book; though sadly, most of us only *move* back and forth from chair to chair. We now move right into my handbook of *Mindful Movement, Where You Are*. These coming pages are by no means any kind of complete or comprehensive encyclopedia of the ways you can incorporate more movement work into your activities of daily living. They're meant instead to be both a challenge and a guide to get you moving and keep you moving and *exploring* ways to develop more and more of your own motion and motivation in your life.

6

Mindful Movement, Where You Are

Explore, or Achieve?

You'll notice how in many of these coming stretching/ awareness/exercise descriptions I'll mention, again and again, the need to remember both to explore instead of achieving *and* to add breath into whatever you're doing. We tend to be an achievement-oriented society. If we can focus on the exploration, with our breath, of our tight and tied places, and **invite that breath and movement** into those places, we can change our world, open our bodies, and even possibly prevent that knee surgery, or hip replacement, or back surgery.

If these concepts appeal to you, I'd recommend finding Egoscue's *Pain Free* book. I think he's made as good a presentation of these ideas as anyone. My earlier book *Meet Your Body* also talks to many of the ideas in this chapter of the book, in a model based on "oiling" the hinges of the body,[1] and *BodymindCORE Work for the Movement Therapist* goes into far more detail about ways to move more effectively and with intention.[2] And Rosenberg's previously mentioned work on the vagus complex feels like the coming wave of learning to get us

---

1   N. Karrasch (2009) *Meet Your Body.* London and Philadelphia: Singing Dragon.
2   N. Karrasch, with R. White and E. Buri (2017) *BodymindCORE Work for the Movement Therapist.* London and Philadelphia: Singing Dragon.

all truly healthy more of the time. All these books can help you if you want more ideas to bring your body back to life.

These exercises work for me because I know my body and its tight and hidden spaces. I've visited them enough to know where I move and where I don't, and I continue to challenge myself to move more freely. My ideas are meant to be a guideline for you, but don't expect to have only my glitches. We each have our individual blueprint and history of aches and pains, traumas and injuries; we must all explore for ourselves. One size does not fit all—a tremendously important concept I wish the allopathic medical community could grasp.

So, **explore letting everything around you be your exercise equipment**. With that primary message, this chapter reaches its conclusions:

- The slower you allow yourself to go as you stretch and work, the more you'll discern and learn about the workings of your body...or the non-workings. Remember, maturity is the ability to discern finer and finer distinctions.

- Realize the same movement ideas will work as well in preparation for your potentially upcoming surgery, and for rehabilitation after surgery has happened and you're working to reclaim your bodymindcore. In the recuperation phase, you'll definitely want to take smaller steps until you've regained your strength.

- Use the rest of this book as/if/when you can to feel stronger and looser.

- The best defense is an offense. You need a bit of movement to melt the tension.

Movement is critical...period. We're all aware of this fact, yet few of us take those steps to keep the body moving and resilient. If you're not yet finding resilience, realize you're in charge of how much movement your body is capable of making, based on how much you challenge it to move. Whether you work out heavily or barely walk across a room: it's critical that you move and keep moving, very possibly moving more than you've been currently been doing.

Let's begin! Each movement described in the coming pages, each awareness I'm asking you to develop, can help you to become more focused in your body, on your problems, in a way that allows you to see if you can really make the positive changes you want. In the back of the book, I'll also give a short summary of which exercises are most effective for which parts of the body or which problems you may face.

SITTING ON THOSE TOES

I invite you to consider that the sitting bones of the pelvis—those two rings called the ischial tuberosities—can be thought of as the feet of the spine. We can sit back on the heels, as most of us do. But we could also choose to sit more "on the toes" of our bottoms. Try it…as you rock back, can you feel your entire spine choose to round and slump, with your head curving forward? As you move towards the front of the sitting bones, it's far harder to slump. Can you feel how much easier it is to sit up straight when you move slightly forward on those sitting bones?

Play with this rocking back and forth motion, making smaller and smaller adjustments until you're just *slightly* on the fronts of these sitting bones. This is your optimal sitting posture in terms of treating the rest of the body correctly. It's just easier to sit here, short term. Yet soon you'll find it takes work to challenge an old habit.

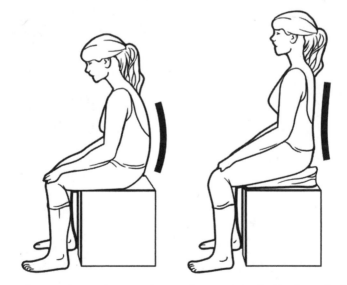

Explore sitting on the toes of sitting bones, instead of back on the heels.

I've often wondered about furniture design. Is there some conspiracy to keep us settled back in our chairs, instead of "on our toes" as we sit? Can we realize we could change our posture just by keeping attention on it? Living with furniture that asks our body to assume an incorrect posture can't be good for us.

And remember how many activities in our daily life involve sitting: driving the car, watching the TV or reading, working in an office or at a computer, craft work—all contribute to that sedentary posture. Even if we can't or won't get out of our seats, can we at least pay attention to the posture of sitting?

A GOOD HEAD ON OUR SHOULDERS

Neckrolls! Shoulder rolls! Too many of us work at computers all day, or drive long hours, or practice detailed craft work. We write, lift or engage in tight and concentrated *effort* of some kind that ties our neck and shoulders in knots. Simply stopping, putting the head upback and on top of the body, then doing slow, smooth neck rolls that explore every single aspect of a backward half circle (or full circle or any part of one) in first one direction, then the other; such a roll can take so much stress out of the head and neck! With different vertebrae of the neck serving as the fulcrum for each bend or roll, and with breath working to reach the areas that have trouble (or pain) accepting breath, you'll often loosen a neck quickly *and* put energy back into the brains. Remember, new theories tell us the brain is present in every cell of our body. Why wouldn't someone sitting at a computer choose to make a few neckrolls every 15 minutes, or half hour? Whether in our "deck chair exercise equipment," a desk chair, a car seat or a dining chair, why not explore more neck movement?

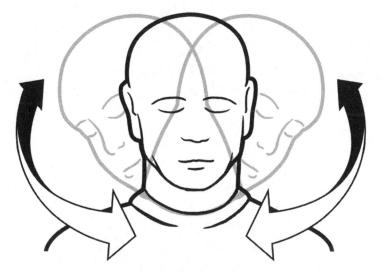

Any seated or standing posture allows for slow and smooth neck rolls from various hinges.

That word "smooth" above is a challenge…most of us have at least one or two places in that circular motion, both neck and shoulders, where some glitch in the circle says "no." Don't curse the glitch! Observe it and invite it to dissolve with your work and your breath. It's never wrong to roll your neck around to try to create space. It seems extreme to me to roll and tax (or jerk and crack!) only the exact same hinge(s) every time you work the neck. Explore; move a bit higher and lower each time. Turn your head slightly further to one side as you roll; try to pull your neck upback as you roll. Find what's angry, listen to it as you breathe.

Too many of us have a "pain in the neck," whether it's a person, a job, an attitude or some past injury that causes us to hold our neck "just so" while holding our breath into our neck, thus never letting breath reach the head. If we can't bring breath and movement into the neck, not only will we never achieve total health, but we also deprive our brain of oxygen by cutting off circulation to the head. Simply rolling the neck around, gently, while breathing and exploring the spots that tell you they don't want to be challenged, lets you know where you need to stretch and move congestion. If you'll gently pay attention to what the neck tells you as you roll around, and make sure breath continues to flow to the neck as you work, you'll be rewarded.

Stanley Rosenberg offers a simple and profound awareness "treatment" in *Accessing the Healing Power of the Vagus Nerve*, and it makes perfect sense. Sit comfortably or lie down. Join your hands with fingers intertwined, then put your hands behind your head. Push your head slightly into your hands, then without turning your head, turn your eyes first to the right for perhaps a minute. You may experience a yawn, or shudder, or deep breath or sigh. Then turn left with your eyes. Whether or not you've found your yawn or other reaction, you've helped to stretch the back of your neck plus many of the muscles and nerves that reside in this area. He believes we can reactivate the ventral vagal system, calming and healing the body. I think you may even reset your own nervous system. How can that be a bad thing?

STILL THE SHOULDERS...

Likewise shoulder rolls...whether sitting or standing, what's so hard about simply lifting your shoulders toward the ceiling, then pulling them straight down toward the floor, then beginning to make circles with those shoulders in a down, forward, up, and back smooth circle? Explore and make it up! Why not send your shoulders into circles together, then opposite each other, in a way that begins moving you in new directions to find your "glitches"?

As I sit, I get one elbow down, out and forward of my body, then use my opposite hand to grab just below that elbow and pull the shoulder out of the ear. Then I bring my occiput (where the head meets the neck) up and back, and find a new and important stretch. I can stretch and draw circles in any direction I explore and find. I intend to create length between elbow and head while breathing deeply. I've been playing with this stretch, and feel progress is again being made.

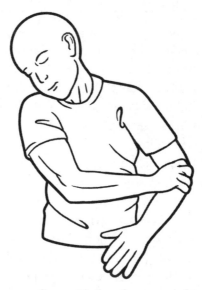

Grab just below one elbow with the other arm and tug mildly, then ask your head and neck to move away, exploring for the stuck spots.

I have a chronic neck injury, with me since I was 3 years old. A car wreck with my grandfather ended up with us sitting in a rolled, upside-down car looking at each other. Since that time my neck has been stiff and tight. Sometimes when I slow down, breathe and roll my neck I can feel myself opening yet another small segment of that injured tissue. I'm not 100 percent released, but my body continues to improve (based at least partly on my desire to continue to maintain and improve), and I'm not giving up on the idea that my neck shouldn't have to remain tight and guarded.

THE CLIMB TO HEALTH IS UP STAIRS

Stairs can be a worthwhile challenge. I realized that several things don't want to happen when I use stairs. First, my right foot doesn't want to contact the step in a straight-on fashion; it likes to point outward as the inner arch lifts off the stair. Simply trying to correct this pattern has already given me a different feeling in the foot, the calf and the body. Next, I realized that I basically still lift myself up the stairs without using toe or ankle hinges… in other words, I simply pull myself up a step without ever using the muscles of the calf which are meant to do most of the work. Often, I allow the arms to help haul me up the steps. While this isn't a bad thing, I'd like to ask the legs to do more of the work.

As I slow my gait and focus on allowing the heel to hang off the edge of the step and sink towards the step below, then lifting up and through that inner arch, I feel a much stronger workout in the calf of that leg. I still experiment with and explore this working of the calf and foot muscles whenever I stop and slow down enough to be aware of my step, on any steps. And when possible, I choose to not use arm railings; working instead to maintain an upright posture while focusing on those feet and leg muscles.

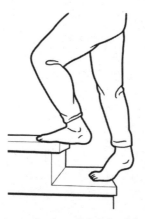

Can you allow your heel to sink below the step, then lift yourself up? Use handrails if needed, but explore this effort.

Perhaps you just can't gather the strength to allow that heel to sink and then lift yourself up onto the step. That's fine! Use those railings and allow your arms to take enough weight so you can find and feel the deep line of the foot and leg you're trying to waken. Like exploring the ability to lift out of a chair while using arms, the development and strengthening of calf muscles for ankle and knee resilience may not happen right away. If you allow yourself to explore these muscles, you have a chance to bring them back into awareness and into movement, and with intention, you may be able to wean yourself from dependence on the arms and transfer some of the work back into the feet and legs.

DOWN STAIRS

Going down stairs is a different challenge. I've realized that, for me, pushups are most difficult when I try to make my body sink back down *slowly*. I decided to add the same idea to descending stairs. So, I focus on really asking my knees to slowly lower my body weight through the descending movement. It's difficult! And again, there's no shame in using the railings for supportive arm strength to assist knees and arches that aren't quite ready for the wakeup call they're being given. Frankly, going down two or three stairs in slow motion will feel like quite a workout the first few times you try...and maybe several times after that as well.

I notice in my own body: my right foot still prefers to turn out as I descend stairs! When I place it straight forward, I feel very different sensations in the knee and leg. I'm reminded of something Ida Rolf is reputed to have said often: "Put it where you want it and ask it to move." Explore.

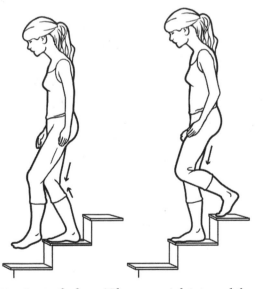

Pay attention to the knees! If you can sink into and through them, they'll begin to feel "oiled" instead of "o l d."

Explore sinking, lengthening *and* lifting the self through the full movement of climbing or descending stairs as well as trying to feel that full movement through the entire body-self. Let's say that another way: Slow down. Mature. Feel every aspect of your foot bed while you remain in tune with the rest of the body as you move up or down stairs. Work to make smoother movement happen in the rest of your body even as you focus on finding each foot and connecting with the stair before moving down to the stairs below.

One doesn't even need to use stairs to experiment with the idea of creating happier knees. Simply standing on one leg, then asking the body to do a one-legged knee bend where you sink into the ground a bit more, will test the limits of your knee and allow you to explore "oiling" that knee hinge. Hold onto a chair or table for balance if necessary. This will also help to make stairs less of a challenge.

SQUATTING: A LOST ART

Many of us complain of knee pain. As with so many other problems, I believe knee pain is another case of "Use it or lose it." For many of us it hurts to squat, so we stop doing it. How can we ever regain use of our knees if we won't try to use them? Sometimes in classes I'll encourage all the students to squat as we begin a course. Many of us are worn out in a matter of minutes, or even seconds—if we can even get there. As with so much in my model, simply slowly paying attention to the movement of squatting can enhance your ability to find well-oiled knees.

One can learn to squat effectively. The previous one-legged knee bending idea is a good beginning, as is paying attention to the knees on stairs. Even if you need to hold onto a chair or table with your hands and arm strength to be able to squat (with either one leg or two), try it. Perhaps you won't be able to keep both feet flat as you squat: perhaps you can't squat at all! I find if I'm squatting for a long period I like to lift one heel slightly while the other foot stays flat as its cylinder carries more weight. I shift back and forth to first one side, then the other, of feet, hips and cylinders. This allows me to stay in squatting posture much longer, thus massaging my knees, hips and back as I squat. As a gardener, this has become my favorite weeding posture.

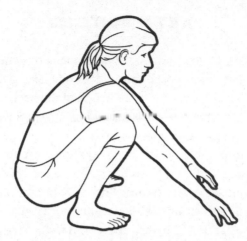

*Squatting is difficult for many of us. Experiment with
this position; possibly keeping one heel at a time off
the ground and shifting from side to side.*

I talked briefly in the segment on the gut area about the
realization that squatting to defecate has advantages. It's also
been shown that cultures that squat more in day to day living
have far fewer problems with backs and knees than our sitting
culture. It's something to think about; we could experiment
with this position more often!

As with everything we've discussed so far, remember this
isn't about achievement but about exploration. Can you allow
yourself to squat even a bit? You may want/need to squat with
arms on a table or counter or while facing an armchair with
your hands on its arms. Take care of yourself. Perhaps the next
time it will be a bit easier…and the time after that…

DON'T BE DE-FEETED!

As you stand in your normal stance, focus on where weight reaches the ground in each foot…does one heel carry most of the weight? Is the weight on the inside of the heel, or outside? How does the other heel respond and react? Does it carry very little weight, or does it carry weight on the opposite edge (inner or outer) from the "heavier" heel? Are you more in your heels or your toes? Do the inner arches sink into the ground, or can you feel yourself nearly pulling them up and off the ground? Now place feet about sitting bone width (not as wide as we often think; more like 10–12 inches apart) and facing straight ahead. Can you approach a clearer balance and explore what it would be like to have your weight sinking into the ground equally through inner and outer heels, inner and outer toes, and inner and outer arches? Could you allow your weight to try to find the entire foot, equally on both sides?

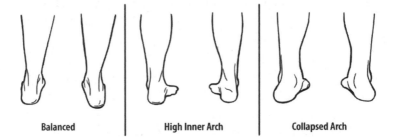

Balanced   High Inner Arch   Collapsed Arch

From left to right: healthy balanced arches; high arches won't touch the ground; flat and fallen arches.

Return to my idea of sitting on the toes of sitting bones instead of on the heels. Can we do the same thing with our feet? Remember the old sayings: "That set me back on my heels." "I'm really feeling on my toes today." Can you see that words describing the activity might influence the attitude and the feeling in the body? Simply stand, find the balance we describe above, then rock slightly forward, then slightly back, and keep rocking back and forth, but making smaller and smaller movements until you land, and stand, slightly in front of your inner arches with a bit more weight in the toes and less in the heels. Remember how we tried the same posture as we sat, and tried to be slightly in front of ourselves? It's a different world when you can stay slightly in your toes.

BIG TOE PUSHUPS

Next, having found the best balance you can realize, explore lifting your body, *using the big toes only*. If the feet and toes still point outward, you'll have a difficult time finding your big toes. Even with feet on straight, chances are you'll realize you lift yourself more into the smaller outer toes than you use the big ones. Work to find that foot straight posture, then slowly lift yourself *through the big toes*, and, even more slowly, come back down onto the ground. Remember that lowering the body weight slowly in a pushup is the hard work. Lowering slowly through big toes is just as hard here as it is in the stair work or in regular face down full body pushups.

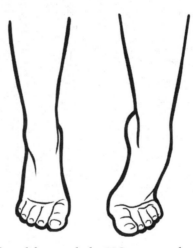

Remember to keep lifting with the BIG toes, not the smaller ones.

After a particularly nasty knee injury (and yes, I'm a Leo, a big cat, and I've used many of my lives!) I found I couldn't lift myself into only my right foot…it simply had no power. As I began big toe pushups to rehabilitate that right leg to trunk line, I found I had to place my arms on a counter or railing, and literally lift myself into the right foot's big toe. Eventually, with enough work and training, I was able to lift myself through the right foot without using arms. Don't be discouraged if you can't do something right away, and don't feel bad if you need "crutches" as you begin working! With a bit of practice, you'll notice positive changes. This is still a difficult exercise for me! Even after years of working with it, because of my wreck injuries my feet don't respond well to the challenge. But the more I work, even when holding onto a table or railing for support, the happier my entire body feels.

I've had several clients tell me they've cured their own plantar fasciitis, and managed to keep it at bay, with a few simple big toe pushups morning and night. And it's so easy to do this, discreetly, anywhere. If I must stand in a line, I'm usually doing mild, slow, subtle toe pushups while I wait. Why not?

BEND AND LIFT?

Remembering the squats, return to knees for a moment: If your knees complain to you quite often, using big toe pushups with slight knee bends at the same time may well give your knees a more flexible sense. Even if you need to hold onto a table or chair for stability, explore big toe pushups *while* using slight knee bends. Slightly flex the knees first, then try that big toe pushup. You'll be rewarded if you stay with the concept.

Now, can you take that toe and ankle flexibility you've just been exploring into more movement? Can you walk with a spring in your step? Many of us shuffle through life, with a "What's the use?" attitude. We have no energy in our feet, our legs, our bodies. If we can explore the toe hinge/toe pushup idea, then translate that hinging and springing action into our walk, life is totally different. Can you explore walking at a slow, steady pace that allows each foot to both sink into the ground, then spring off through the toes, instead of shuffling through life?

I've visited Jamaica often, and taught bodywork classes there, mostly for US massagers. Often, I'll point out, and the group will observe, the walk of native Jamaicans on the beach. They have a saunter that's not seen in many of our "Westernized" cultures. Most Americans and Europeans walk down the beach like they're on a life-or-death mission to somewhere: head forward, possibly down, and achieving distance. They miss the scenery and rarely stop to enjoy the beauty they've come to see. It's a joke to me: They're walking so fast through paradise that they totally miss it.

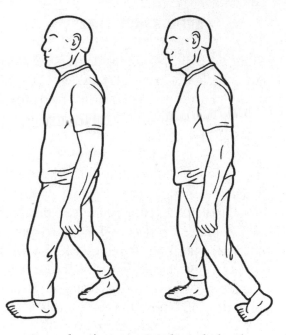

*Pretend you're sauntering down the beach,
not rushing to an appointment.*

Jamaicans, on the other hand, seem to allow each step to take its proper time. Their feet seem to sink into the ground, grasp it, and then spring off from it. It looks (and feels) almost effortless compared to what I see most Westerners doing when they walk on the beach. I'd encourage you to walk with this concept: Stroll. Saunter. Sink in/push off and stroll/saunter/sink in/push off. If you try this walk, can you feel a difference? Particularly if you challenge yourself to push off with your toes and have that spring in your step, I think you'll feel a difference, possibly all the way up into your back and shoulders. After exploring, go back to your old way of walking. Do you feel that difference? Which do you prefer? Many folks on returning to their old way of walking realize it hurts their low back when they're heavy in the heels. That should get most of us excited about relearning how to walk happily.

BEND, TWIST, FLEX

Bending: Sadly, too many of us don't do it! If we won't oil the hinges of our spine, how will they stay resilient? Why shouldn't a disc herniate, or bulge? We could benefit greatly from simple forward and backward bends. Reach gently towards toes and unwind the spine downforward, segment by segment. Then straighten back up and continue into a backward bend, extending the spine in the other direction: This stretch can be an amazing rejuvenator.

Please note I'm not suggesting you must either touch your toes or be able to make a perfect backward crescent moon in your extended open position. Take yourself to a comfortable exploration, not an agonizing achievement. If your achievement takes your breath away, you're too deep and too fast. Back off, breathe, and stretch only until you're able to keep breathing into the stretch. Again, explore slowing the movement, trying to find each vertebra of the spine as you move the spine forward and backward, and breathe into each spinal segment as you move.

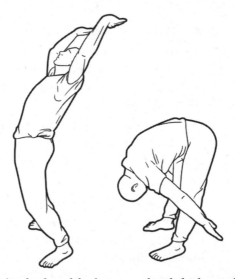

The further back and forth you can bend, fairly comfortably, the healthier and happier your spine will become.

Chances are, like most of us, you won't be able to isolate or "feel" each segment. Most of us have a section of mid to low back where a whole group of vertebrae "jumps" forward or back…we simply can't isolate and use individual hinges. Many of us have an entire segment in the upper back that seems permanently fixed into a forward roll position. Too often we don't try to find such hinges to ask for slightly more movement each time we bend or flex. **Play with this forward and back hinge work in the spine**, and you'll feel the reward in many ways. Chances are you'll feel fewer neck and head problems, a freer back, better posture and, possibly, even happier feet and legs.

I'll even work to "open the heart hinge" by lying down with a pillow underneath the most prominent curved part of my spine…right around my heart. Simply asking that section of spine to lay over the pillow, open forward, with breath, can enhance standing posture and make you feel freer.

TWIST AND TURN

In addition to forward and back bending, other directions of movement add resilience to the body. Experiment with twisting the spine/upper body left and right. Use your arms as liberally or sparingly as your body tolerates, but think of moving your arms in all directions, primarily on the twisting side to side plane. My arms and hands begin and sometimes stay at my sides at shoulder height. I use three to five pound weights as I twist and try to bring my visual focus 180 degrees behind me, anchoring on the same spot from both directions. Weights aren't needed! They're something I add, but simply moving the body parts through space and thereby slowly twisting fascial networks will accomplish the movement needed.

And remember, this twisting can even be done without weights and in the comfort of a deck or other chair. Why not simply sit in an arm chair as you watch TV: Put both hands on one arm of the chair and twist, hold still and breathe. Then return to center and move to the other side.

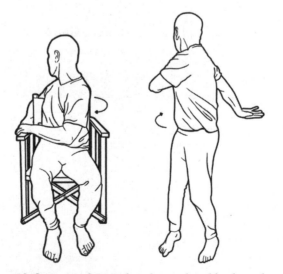

As with flexing and extending forward and backward,
twisting movements will also increase spinal flexibility.

I work slowly, exploring my entire body and monitoring to keep all parts engaged. In my own body, as I stand and twist to the right, my right inner arch wants to leave the floor. It's an interesting extra challenge to notice such subtle movement, flatten and re-anchor the tightened arch, breathe and keep working.

I truly believe if we'd all just spend a bit of time each day with bending forward and backward, twisting our entire body side to side, and flexing laterally or to the side (see Side Flexion on next page), we'd be stretching so much of the body with simple movements. What's stopping us?

SIDE FLEXION

With a lateral, side to side flexion, bend to one side, then the other. The more you keep your entire body, including arms in a straight plane/line in side posture as you lean to first one side, then the other, the more you create a true lateral flexion and the more you ask the spine to find yet another pattern of stuck places that want to release. I like using a mirror to visually check on my body's line when I'm side bending. Monitoring my body helps me isolate the pieces that want to "cheat" in that movement. I also realize that, by reaching higher with my "long" arm, I stretch shoulder muscles that would rather stay unstretched.

It's interesting to "think global while acting local" with this and all the ideas I present. As you move entirely to one side, pay attention to the opposite footbed—does all or part try to leave the ground? What changes when you try to keep the feet anchored evenly as you move? Attention to these details can make your stretching more productive.

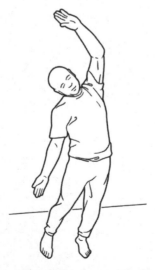

Staying on a long and straight plane while flexing side to side can also increase spinal function and enhance health.

My spine no longer moves easily since it was fused from T10 to L3 in 1987. Even so, I visualize myself bending to the side, and making wavy undulations, somewhat like a snake or belly dancer. It doesn't truly happen, but I can imagine more and more flexibility is coming back into my body, and, when I do, I feel better. And in terms of my "fused" spine, it's much more flexible than that of most 69-year-old people I know!

NOW FOR THE DRIVERS...

Think about those who must drive often—perhaps you're one of them. I've seen many clients come to me with left sciatic pain. I'll usually ask right away if they drive much, and many do so. In my model, when a person drives a lot, they sit in or on the right sitting bone more as they overuse the right foot for the gas and brake pedals. The left sitting bone doesn't quite reach the car seat. For me, this suggests jamming the right deep spinal muscle, the psoas, which runs from the inside of the leg to the front of the spine, into a shortened and tight configuration. The body's left side has then shortened its antagonist muscles to counterbalance.

The iliacus, inside the hipbone to the inside of the leg, and the quadratus lumborum, which begins at the top of the hipbone and reaches up to the twelfth rib and spinal bones, tighten to hold the other side of this pattern in place. When that deep front-of-spine psoas on the right side gets tight, those deep hip/back muscles, iliacus and quadratus, on the left respond and pull their hip short and tight, causing an impingement of the left sciatic nerve. It's common sense: if something gets too tight nd something else decides to hold on to help, then everybody's unhappy.

I'll often try to shift more of my weight into the left side of my body while driving. I pretend I can make the left sitting bone push further into the seat than the right bone will push. And I move around quite a bit when I drive. I'll also shift which spinal hinge contacts the seat back most.

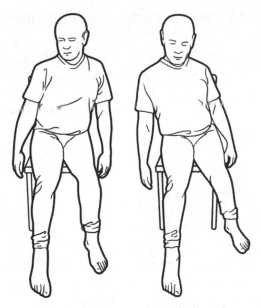

Shifting the weight on long drives can lessen back and sciatic problems.

Simple attention to posture in driving, plus taking short breaks more frequently, moving around and shifting weight from side to side while driving, shifting the seat in all directions—these things can help someone keep their own sciatic pain at bay. And, as always, I'm not suggesting one achieves, as much as explores patterns, keep breath in the picture and observe self and patterns to make changes in them.

I remember one client who had to drive a great deal for his work. He self-maintained by coming to see me every 6000 miles, for his maintenance and "tune-up." Can you develop such awareness, that you know when you need to stop and go?

OPENING THE SACROILIAC JUNCTIONS

Too often, whether it's due to too much driving, too much sitting in general, holding onto the pelvic floor, or any of many other reasons, our sacroiliac junctions get tied into seeming knots. We'll get a pain down one side of the back or the other; possibly a sciatic issue of pain or numbness shooting down one leg. Simply working to open and "oil" these sacroiliac (SI) junctions can reduce the pain and irritation of the tension in the hip and leg region.

Explore: Lie on your back, on the floor or a bed. Think of lengthening one heel and leg as far from your hips as you can move it. At the same time, jam the second leg up into yourself, keeping the leg and knee straight and short. Hold this posture for several breaths. Then relax, breathe again, and shift the legs so that the "shorter" leg becomes the longer and the longer now jams into its hip. Explore back and forth, asking the SI junctions to lengthen, open and find space.

Clearly this stretch, along with the hamstring stretches to come, can help with sciatic issues. And as too many of us sit too long and too much of the time, this can be a simple aid to opening the clogged SI and hip areas.

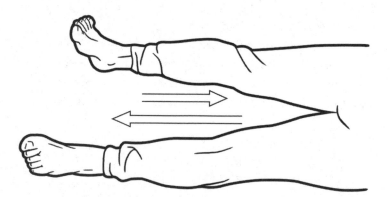

Simply shift your legs so one is long and one is jammed; while breathing, give attention to finding energy in the hips and groin.

Too many of us have low back and sciatic pains...some because we drive too much; some because we sit too much, cross our legs mostly in one direction, and so on. Work to stay open in the hip and SI region can make the entire body feel better: knees, feet and hips, but even the trunk and shoulders, can benefit from staying loose in the hip region. Using this stretch and breath work in addition to the hamstring stretches below can help many problems of the hips, low back, sciatic nerve and sometimes even into the legs as well as the mid back. Explore.

UNDERTHINGS: HAMSTRINGS AND ADDUCTORS

Hamstrings! Adductors! I tend to believe that, right in the junction of the groin on each leg, the inner hamstrings and adductor muscles end up shortening, tightening and gluing to each other, just where they attach to bones. Many of us grip our pelvic floor too tightly. How do we unwind this area, which I think are the "gird your loins" muscles?

Adductor stretches can help: Lie on your back and bring your knees up so your feet are flat on the floor. Then simply allow knees (and feet) to fall out to the side, comfortably. While observing where they fall open and where they decide they won't (with breath and allowing gravity to take them a bit further), you can begin to release the adductors deep inside the upper thighs, and also to stretch the hamstrings, especially the inner ones.

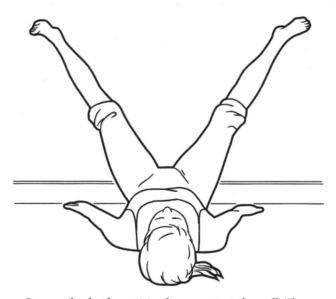

On your back, place sitting bones against the wall. Then allow the legs to slowly sink and open to the sides.

To make this stretch more challenging, lie face down but try to spread the knees in the same movement as the "falling open" posture. Not an easy stretch!

A more difficult adductor stretch invites you to lie on the floor with sitting bones up against a wall and feet/legs reaching towards the ceiling on the wall. Then simply allow the legs to open and reach out and toward the floor.

HAMSTRINGS ALONE

For the very important hamstrings we have several good techniques. The first I've already described…forward bends. If focusing on hamstrings, however, instead of really working to find individual spinal segments as you move forward, now focus on finding those muscles on the back of the thighs, right up into the hips. To make this even more delicious, while standing and bending, face a wall and stand about 12–18 inches from it. Allow the back of your head to slide down the wall *while* turning the toes of the feet to the inside—a pigeon-toed position as you bend forward. Chances are you'll really feel the extra inner hamstring stretch from this simple turning in of feet. And, if you'll keep your inner arches anchored to the floor, you'll find even more stretch through the body, especially the hamstrings. Remember, breath is always good!

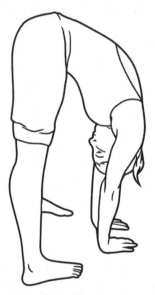

The more you can bend forward, the better the stretch, especially if you can keep feet pointed inside and inner arches on the ground. If you have trouble reaching this position, consider using an armchair for support: hands on chair arms and head reaches towards the seat.

When I travel and don't have time, space or equipment to work out or stretch, I try to use this simple (not easy!) stretch for 90 seconds each morning in the shower cabinet or against a wall. I find the more I remain pigeon-toed *while* tugging my head down the wall *while* keeping my low back up and inner arches down, the more I feel the stretch on the inner hamstrings. Can you find a different focus: bottom, middle and top of the hamstrings?

AN EASIER HAMSTRING STRETCH

You can also get a satisfying hamstring stretch by using a belt or stretching strap, lying on your back, and bringing one leg up into a 90-degree posture—leg straight toward the ceiling. Put that strap or belt across the transverse arch of the foot—right at the middle of the foot—then tug mildly taking the foot toward your head (*while* you keep your hip on the floor), until you begin to feel that stretch/possibly burn. The burn indicates you're asking fascial restrictions (the connective tissue that wraps muscles and runs through them) to unwind. A little burn is good; a lot is probably too much. As with all these stretches, chances are you didn't get tight hamstrings in five minutes, so you may want to make this an ongoing exploration instead of a quick fix. Holding one leg in the air, with the belt or strap allowing you to hold the posture, you can release hamstring tension and make a low back feel much freer as well. Remember again: Breath is critical! If you can't find a full breath at the top of a stretch, I believe you're stretching too far.

As I stretch hamstrings on clients, I often encourage them to see hamstrings and low back muscles as one continuous stream of muscle tissue. I suggest the sitting bones (ischial tuberosities) are the pulleys of this longer muscle combination. Usually, I can stretch hamstrings for a client in a way that allows them to feel the connection between hamstrings and low back muscles.

I also like exploring foot positions, and directions of the leg's turning while I stretch. Simply turn the foot inside and outside or bring big or small toes closer into the body, or turn the knee in and out: All these small movements can change the way the hamstrings *and* the back feel while you stretch.

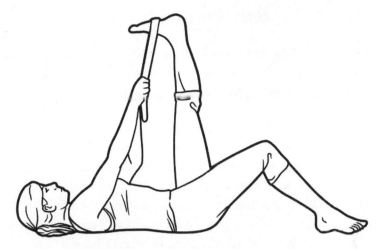

A straight-legged hamstring stretch, using a belt or strap and common sense, will allow you to stretch both hamstrings and lower back at the same time.

While many therapists would argue with me, I prefer to keep the legs straight and the knees nearly locked when I stretch hamstrings. I understand that damage can be done, but I feel if one uses that good old common sense and monitors breath, one can find exactly how far to stretch that straight leg to accomplish the most release.

ARMS: THE FRONT LEGS

Too many of us don't think about upper body strength or conditioning…I'm one of those. However, one of my favorite stretches involves lengthening and decompressing the arms—literally, pulling them out of the shoulder sockets a bit. To that end, I'll often find a doorway with solid overhead trim where I can place my fingers at the top of the trim, then allow the rest of my body to hang off the doorway. I might also use an outside deck that allows me to reach a solid platform from which to hang. Anything you can find as exercise equipment that allows you to hang from your hands will open shoulder girdles and arms. Think about it: When we hang from our hands, arms and shoulders, for the first time our spine is being stretched and straightened and *hung from the shoulders* instead of our shoulders hanging from our spine. How could this be a bad thing?

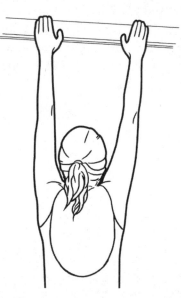

Hanging from the doorway or some higher perch allows the spine to fall out of the shoulders instead of the shoulders hanging from the spine. Experiment with one-armed hanging, with a twist.

As you "hang around" in this posture, experiment with twists and turns…explore, find parts of the shoulder girdle that complain, use one arm only and listen to the complaints! Don't decide to overpower the complainers; just allow them to speak to you, listen and honor what they have to say to you. Chances are they'll stop shouting so loudly if you just stop and listen.

HANGING FROM THE FRONT LEGS

A true bar such as a chin-up bar is probably a better piece of equipment in terms of ability to grasp and hang than a doorway trim or deck, but use what equipment is before you. I've never had great arm strength, but I'm finding that simply putting my hands on a railing, a counter, a table or desk and lifting my upper body with my upper arms can help me stretch and lengthen the spine nearly as well…with the added bonus of calling on a bit of strength in those arms. Pull ups are still beyond my expertise; that doesn't mean I don't still give them a try every now and then. One day I'll be surprised! I see arms as front legs and would like to have strength in all my legs, not just the back ones.

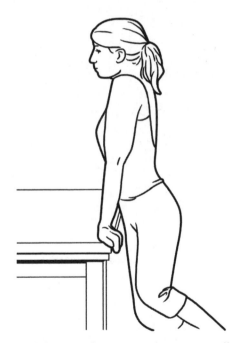

As with hanging from arms, this position allows you to let your spine hang freely from your shoulders instead of the shoulders hanging from the spine.

I've mentioned earlier the "that which we have" concept of using what's around me as exercise equipment. Thus, a railing, table, counter, back of couch or whatever is in front of you can provide support and assist in this stretch.

Remember this concept: Instead of hanging your arms from your spine, you're now hanging your spine off your shoulders. Think how this invites your body to assume new positions and create awareness in new spots. You might even hear a few spinal bones release "something" as you hang around. Realize you're inviting the upper body to open, breathe and relax as you ask it to awaken.

WRISTS AND FINGERS TOO

One last idea for arms and shoulders: Wrists and fingers can get too tight; carpal tunnel issues, arthritis in the finger joints, trigger fingers or thumbs, de Puytren's syndrome, and so on. What to do? So many simple things can be done if we only take the time! Why not practice rolling the hands/wrists around as we did with the neck, taking the fingers first as far upback as we can get them before rolling the hands in circles, thus stretching wrists as we'd stretch ankles? Why not explore taking the fingers of one hand and pulling the fingers of the other hand back towards the body, with breath? How can we truly expect our hands to be happy if we primarily keep the fingers tight and flexed? Simply remembering to move them into a more open posture can make great progress in keeping them free.

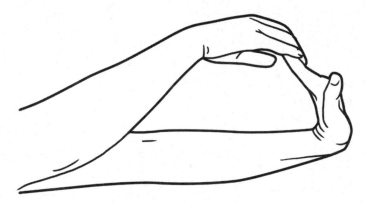

*Can you see how we don't often challenge the
fingers to find an opposite motion?*

Use it or lose it—trite but true. Several years ago, my fingers began to feel "arthritic" from so much deep bodywork I was giving to others; I abused my fingers. I simply began massaging and stretching them; I'm good for another 10,000 miles!

You've already heard my concept of hands as front feet and arms as front legs. We'll return to this next, but consider that, anatomically, hands and feet both have arches, five digits, "heels," plantar/palmar surfaces and bones beyond ankle and wrist that anchor most of the muscles that extend all the way down into feet and hands. The similarities are interesting and, once you see them, you can see why we'd like to get more movement into front feet as well as back ones.

ANIMAL WALKS

Put these last ideas together: Working to free hands, wrists and fingers as well as elbows and shoulders, suggests we might want to experiment with walking on all fours. I've long thought we should spend a bit more time on our front feet, legs and hips (the hands, arms and shoulders). To that end, I'll get into a pushup position, try to keep a flat and open back, and walk across an open space on four legs. Usually I'll start with a "tiger walk" which brings one hand and opposite leg moving together. Then I'll move on to a "bear walk" which allows same side hand and foot to move together. Hard work!

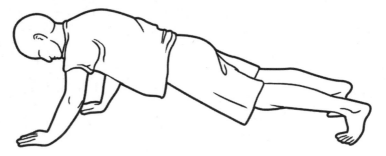

In addition to exploring horizontal animal walks, can you even try putting your weight in different parts of your "front feet"?

Now, to make this even more interesting, why not experiment with shifting the placement of the footbed of those front legs? In other words, where in your hand does the weight touch the ground? Can you change it? Can you explore to see which parts of your hands don't feel like connecting to the ground? Chances are it will be the fingers/toes…interesting that most of us also put more weight through the heels of our feet as well as through the palms/heels of our hands. Can you challenge yourself to move from different parts of your front feet as you walk around on all fours?

This is one of the more difficult ideas I'm offering in this section of the book, so don't be discouraged if you can't master such a walk. When this exercise was first suggested to me by a chiropractor friend, it was all I could do to take three steps in this posture before being totally worn out and unable to continue. It took much of the summer for me to learn to make 30 steps—ten tiger, ten bear, ten more tiger. By the end of the summer, however, my back felt better than it had felt in years! It's all related...

BACK ON OUR TOES

I'd like to return to the feet and toes for just a moment. Perhaps this idea makes more sense in terms of recuperating from a surgery; but it's actually something to pay attention to all the time. There's a tremendous correlation between what goes on in the feet and what happens in the body everywhere above.

The first time I truly understood this truth, I was exploring the joints in my big toe. As I literally "cranked" my big toe underneath my foot, then tried to make circles with it, something in my neck snapped! Nothing was happening in my neck at the time; it was totally brought on by the movement of my big toe. This got me thinking…

I believe if we'd all pay more attention to creating movement and resilience in the entire footbed, but specifically in the toes themselves, we'd feel much freer all through the body. Think of this: At any time, but especially after a surgery, can you see how just rubbing the soles of the feet and trying to create a bit more flexibility in the toes could help your entire body?

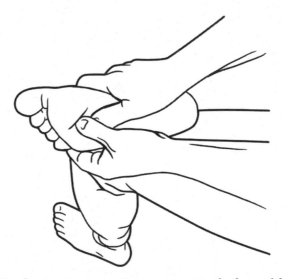

Simple attention to creating movement in the feet and footbeds
can bring movement, energy and health above as well.

Why not sit around, before or after a surgery, and simply hold one foot in your hands (if your body will reach that far), then both rub deeply and slowly on the plantar surface, or bottom, of your foot? Why not take that big toe and move it around, imagining you can "oil" that joint? Can you see how simply working with that foot could improve flexibility up and down the body?

There's a spot in the foot, between the big toe and second toe, and right where the bones of the two toes join, that's called Bubbling Spring or Bubbling Well in acupuncture and Chinese medicine work. If we can learn to massage this (what I call the "Be Well" spot), I think we'll stay healthier all through the body.

If you're not able to reach your own foot (whether because of surgery pain or just inflexibility issues) could someone do a bit of foot rubbing for you? You may be amazed both at how good much of footwork feels, but also how sore a few spots can be. Any reflexology chart can show you a roadmap of which parts of the foot's sole correlate to organs, bones and regions above. As long as you remain in charge, telling your partner whether the pressure is too little, too much or just right, they'll be helpful.

Sometimes you can't reach your own foot and there's no one around to help you. Find a tennis ball or something of roughly that resilience and texture; roll around on that ball for a minute or two as you stand on the other foot (or even sit), place a bit of weight onto the ball, then roll. I've seen quite a few clients who keep backs happier with a bit of this simple rolling of the plantar surface. Try it!

The earliest I ever worked on a client after surgery was two hours! I went to visit a friend in hospital right after her hysterectomy and spent about 20 minutes gently rubbing her feet. She claimed later that I was a "lifesaver." As long as any footwork is done gently and soothingly, I don't see a problem with working reasonably quickly after most surgeries.

AN ALL PURPOSE CUE

One last simple—not easy!—idea will be offered as I close this chapter: I believe if we could all learn to live our lives with our belly button held back into the stomach while our head fits up and back, it would enhance our posture, alleviate much back pain, enhance digestion and elimination functions and even make the head and neck feel better! So please, take away from this and every section the concept of keeping the waist back and head on top, no matter what you're doing in any moment.

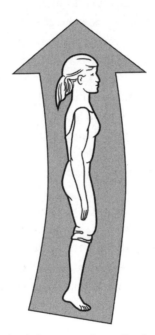

Head up, waist back, heart out front, flex knees and breathe!

I've realized that, due to the back pain I have most days, each time I get up I remain in a slightly fetal posture, with head and shoulders forward. As I realize this posture has become my habit, I now explore breaking that habit. So, every time I stand, I take a moment to "put a good head on my shoulders." I often talk to clients about thinking of themselves as being the general who watches and directs the battle from above and afar instead of being the foot soldier who might just get his head blown off his body! It's a great image: Can you see yourself as having a head that lives upback above your body instead of running interference out front so much of the time?

Add one more thought to the idea above…What if your heart was the first segment of your body to arrive in any situation? Do you see how most of us "hide our hearts" and droop into a slumped posture? If we could keep head up, waist back and heart out front, what a truly wonderful world we could enjoy!

In my earlier book *Freeing Emotions and Energy Through Myofascial Release*,[3] I introduce my head/heart/gut/groin model to clients who want to improve their flexibility. I suggest if we'd just learn to keep head, heart, gut and groin centers both further apart and in a straighter line, much of what causes poor health wouldn't have a place to slow down and congest our bodies into illness. In my later book *BodyMindCORE Work for the Movement Therapist*, I further add to the model by suggesting strictures or gateways between these four centers as well as between the ground and groin and between the head and heavens. If we could pay attention to our four centers and these five gateways and work to keep our body longer and in straighter alignment, I'm not sure we'd need doctors nearly as much as we think we do. Add the extremities from this book, and you have a pretty good picture of how I think we stay well: keep head, heart, gut and groin open and allow energy to move into and through the extremities, with resilience. Simple, not easy…

I hope, from this *Mindful Movement* chapter, you've gained ideas that will let you see how you can be more mindfully active without having to alter too much of your life. Simple attention to how we sit, stand, walk and work…mindful movement makes sense. What do you have to lose, other than some aches,

---

3   N. Karrasch (2012) *Freeing Emotions and Energy Through Myofascial Release.* London and Philadelphia: Singing Dragon.

maybe some pounds and some potential health challenges that are lurking closer when you don't pay attention to your bodymindcore?

In the past, I also wanted to title one of my books *Now: Do Something!* A student, working on me in a bodywork session and knowing I believed in breath and movement to accompany the work, couldn't decide what movement to ask for and gave that instruction. I laughed, and that helped her achieve what she needed. It's true! You don't go wrong with that piece of advice. I second the motion: Now: Do Something!

So, the first part of this book is finished. We've discussed how a balanced lifestyle and attitude can bring you to health or at least help you to retrieve some part of it. In this coming part you'll find my suggestions for the three stages of surgery: preventing, preparing for and recovering from and rebuilding after surgery has taken place. Chances are one section of the three is on your mind more just now…you may be tempted to jump right to that section, and that will work. Do consider that the five elements of this first part suggest the need to be in balance, the information from the various sections joins together to offer ideas to support general health. So, I hope you'll look at all the chapters. Let's go ahead!

Part II

SURGERY!

The three main chapters of this second part are devoted to three goals: how to prevent surgery from becoming necessary, how to prepare yourself if surgery becomes inevitable, and how to recuperate, recover and repair more quickly and fully from any surgery. I hope the ideas will resonate with you and inspire you to get up and take the steps needed to make your life healthier. As I've said before, I've not done everything correctly or well in my journey, but I have seen each step as a learning process, and I'd like to share what I've learned so you don't have to fall into the same holes I've found along the road.

I've invited my friend Dan Kuebler, also a health care professional, with another perspective on surgery, to join in with his thoughts, which serve as a springboard for me to also talk about some important points. And I've asked Ralph Harvey, MD, a family practice doctor and my brother-in-law and colleague in wellness for many years, to write a few words to close each section—sort of a "last opinion from the doc." Feel free to spend more time on the section that closely follows where you are on the path, but realize the entire book has good ideas to keep you on the road to optimal health. So, let's begin with tips to keep surgery at bay.

Our Thoughts Are Prayers

Our thoughts are prayers, and we are always praying...
Our thoughts are prayers, take charge of what you're saying.
Seek a Higher consciousness, a state of peacefulness,
And know that God is always there
And every thought becomes our prayer.

Lucille Olson, Lansing, Michigan

7

Preventing a Surgery

DAN'S STORY

As a practicing physical therapist of 40 years I never, ever saw myself as having something physically go wrong with my body that would stop me from doing what I wanted to do. I was an athlete, an organic market gardener for 28 years. I could toss my grandkids high in the air, could ballroom dance the night away, and could captain sail boats and sail the Caribbean. In my world, physical disease and injury only happened to others, not to me.

Sure, there were many old athletic injuries when I was younger. A ruptured Achilles tendon, a traumatic multiple fracture to my right leg when a child of 7 on the school playground's merry-go-round, multiple sprained ankles during high school and college basketball, and even the occasional fall from horses: Eventually these injuries convinced me I wasn't immortal. However, in youth all is possible, and all these little injuries seemingly healed so I was able to go on my way...that is, until around my 60th year.

My trouble started very gradually with a mildly sharp, small pain in my right groin area upon standing after I'd been driving/sitting in the car for 30–60 minutes at a time (and as a traveling physical therapist, I spent plenty of time in the car!). Since it didn't always happen, I paid little attention to this small discomfort. **I went** on my way for years, and only in hindsight realized I began to gradually compensate in my daily motions and activities to protect the irritated area from undue pressure. I was an active guy, and I did what I had to do to get my work done.

This pattern continued for another 2–3 years, but with the slow addition of soft tissue and muscle tenderness creeping into the mix of symptoms, and nocturnal leg discomfort at times, I had to pay attention. Of course, being a physical therapist, I self-diagnosed my problem as "tensor fascia lata syndrome" and began working on stretches and pressure point therapy as well as working with several myofascial practitioners. Symptoms would decrease after many of these sessions, but unfortunately relief was only temporary, for a day or two at best. As part of this exploratory process I found myself also looking into several alternative approaches. Among the avenues I explored: acupuncture, massage, fascial release and Egoscue movement method. I was faithful to the stretches/awareness/exercises given to me, but eventually I realized I couldn't get ahead of the debilitating pain. I did what I knew how to do, and I couldn't keep the pain at bay. Sadly, it was time to move forward.

Relax!

In each of these three chapters and scenarios we'll first talk about remembering to relax. It's so easy to allow yourself to get worked up and visualize a worst-case scenario. Can you allow yourself instead to take your breath, relax and remind yourself that others have managed to prevent surgeries, and very possibly you can and will do as well? Can you allow yourself to realize also that you can invest in higher-quality lifestyle choices (more vitality in movement, healthier diet, mindful emotional health, slower and deeper breathing and social connectedness) to better your chances of *not* needing the surgery many people accept "just because they've gotten older and fallen apart"? Did Dan's words above describing his process, resonate for you?: "only in hindsight (I) realized I began to gradually compensate in my daily motions and activities to protect the irritated area from undue pressure." The information is there; too many of us choose to avoid noticing it. Perhaps he simply forgot that tiny but profound word "relax."

▌ I don't think health is achieved—I think it's discovered.

Relaxation isn't easy, but it's possible. We're hearing more and more about people who've realized they've worked themselves into constant pressures; they've become task-rich and quality-time poor. The simplest *and* hardest task I can give a client or friend is to ask them to relax! Often, I'll suggest to a client "OK, you're an achiever…today I challenge you to learn to *achieve relaxation.* I'd like you to put on a CD, lie on the floor and listen to one or two songs all the way through. Don't do anything but keep your mind still and focus on breath and relaxation. Don't sort the mail, don't make lists in your head, and don't think of anything but breath and relaxation for one or two whole songs. Can you *achieve* that?" I don't think health is achieved—I think it's discovered. If that's so, it makes more sense to learn to explore than to try to manage the journey. But—that *achiever* may need a goal to be able to find the way to relaxation.

Following that thought: Often a client will ask some form of this question at the end of a bodywork session. Their query will be a variation of "Is it all right if I (swim, run, work out, do yoga or tai chi, go back to work) now? My answer is simple: "It depends…can you go into the activity in *exploration mode*, or will you have to achieve?" If you can allow yourself to *explore* the workout, the yoga, the workplace, it's fine to go back to your activity. But if you feel the need to achieve, you've lost the ground you just gained. Relax, explore, heal.

Years ago, one of my mentors came to my town and presented a workshop. After, our parked car windshield had been targeted with a flyer for a "stress reduction" workshop. My mentor looked at the flyer and said, "I have a two-word answer to stress: So what?" This was before the "don't sweat the small stuff/it's all small stuff" line was going around. Both sentiments are correct. Stressing about what you may or may not have control over seems a poor way to stay healthy. My grandfather, who lived to 93 and whom I emulate, used to tell us: "One hundred years from now, that won't matter at all." That was around 60 years ago, and he's correct already.

What You Focus On, Expands

Can we prevent surgeries? Absolutely! First, let's note that various studies have shown that many placebo surgeries seem to provide as much relief as the "real" ones, whether it be with meniscus tears in the knees, low back issues or even gall bladder removals. Other studies show that many people with no back pains or problems exhibit compressed discs or pinched nerves in their backs. Thus, if you have back problems, chances are good the surgeon will find something to "fix" even if it's not actually the true cause of your problem. Common sense suggests that if we move, stretch fascial restrictions and continue to "oil" our machinery, it will work for us longer and better. We can't prevent every surgery with attitude, breath, water and movement, but we can prevent many, if we'll try.

I recall Larry Dossey's book, *Healing Words*.[1] Dossey, a scientist and surgeon, set out to review the literature of scientific experiments dealing with the effectiveness of prayer on healing. I believe he thought he'd be able to prove that prayer wasn't actually very important in the healing equation. After reviewing something over 100 studies about prayer and healing, he found a great majority of these studies pointed to the realization that prayer was a factor in enhancing healing. Prayer is energy... when plants were receiving good energy or thoughts (prayers),

---

1   L. Dossey (1993) *Healing Words*. New York: Harper Collins.

they thrived more than plants that received no energy, or had bad energy directed towards them. Some studies were simple, where scientists gave attention to one set of plants and ignored another; some were double-blind hospital studies where the prayer team prayed for a person unknown to them. Nearly all these studies showed prayer to be effective.

Most interesting to me: Dossey found that the very most effective prayer one could use was simply "Thy will be done." I'm fascinated that he realized taking the ego and its desire to control out of the prayer made prayer more effective, immediately. Since reading this book many years ago, I've made more effort to allow the Universe to handle the details for me. I still work and strive to move in a positive direction, but I'll also let myself relax, coast, and assume a Higher Power knows what I need and wants to restore me to perfect health…if I can just assist by getting out of my own way! I remember a prayer group who opened their weekly meetings by singing "Row, row, row your boat, gently down the stream; merrily, merrily, merrily, merrily, life is but a dream." That's actually a pretty good little metaphysical hymn, isn't it?

Years ago a student gave me a small purple business card. It simply said, "Dear _____, I don't need your help today. Thank you very much. Love, God." Too many of us try to control the Universe instead of flowing in it. Years ago, I wrote a song: "Are you gonna row, or are you gonna flow?" It makes more sense to go with the tide and enjoy the ride. I've always returned to the idea that a power higher than mine probably has a perfect answer if I can get out of the way and allow that power to manifest in my life.

Many of us would prefer a life where all is predictable and same…we don't like surprises. To some degree we all want to control the entire Universe and the workings in it; the truth is, this isn't possible. None of us has control of the Universe, and there will be surprises and disappointments along our journey. By being open to a highest good and praying for that good instead of being specific in what you want your world to look like, you're less likely to limit the power of the Universe. A line I often end my prayer thinking with is simply "This, or something better, Father."

If you're a pray-er, continue your prayer work and invite those you love and trust to join you. If you don't subscribe to a religious pattern, you can still visualize, affirm, see life and light flowing through your being, and in general intend for health and healing to come into your world, your body, and your environment. Whether you call it prayer or positive affirmation or attitude, it's effective. And remember, the less your thoughts involve directing the Universe to your way of thinking, the more effective it's likely to be. The more you pray in positive gratitude instead of negative mindset about your lack or need, the more your reward tries to find you, and more quickly.

> To some degree we all want to control the entire Universe and the workings in it; the truth is, this isn't possible. By being open to a highest good and praying for that good instead of being specific in what you want your world to look like, you're less likely to limit the power of the Universe.

I've always felt Lucille Olson tapped into a piece of wisdom with the song that opened Part II. What you focus on expands. Are you focusing on the positive aspects of your life and health, or do you choose to worry and be fearful about what could go wrong?

Besides focusing on the positive, how do the Type As, the tightly wound, the achievers…how do they/we achieve relaxation? It's hard. If you haven't tried yoga, or meditation, either might be a helpful path. If you're secure in your church and religion, you already know that getting into a prayerful state, alone and with others, can induce that relaxation as you find a feeling of sanctuary as well, and that having faith in the goodness of your God reassures that all will work for the highest good. But with or without that faith, if you want to change this achieving, feeling-frayed habit, what can you do for yourself?

I'd suggest nature as a prayerful, meditative and relaxing and therefore positive experience. Whether taking nice walks, working in the garden, watching the movement of clouds, or even simply keeping one or two herbs on your windowsill and admiring the sun and clouds outside the window—even if only for a second or two—you can find ways to allow nature to interact with you; seek to observe and be soothed by it.

Relaxing into life and accepting what it offers is important! I've often thought that *relaxation* and *recreation* are simply abilities to concentrate on something other than your normal activities and thoughts. A continued state of laxity *or* creativity is good if not driven to extremes. Relaxation or recreation may be pleasure reading instead of work reading or study; listening to music or enjoying television instead of feeling you need to be productive. Relaxation or recreation could come from physical activity or volunteer service or from socializing with friends or taking that nature walk. For me, the most effective restoration comes from working in my garden and yard, especially when I can remember to disengage from the achievement mode and simply relax and enjoy the work without setting challenges to achieve everything in one day.

To relaxation and recreation, I'll add one more important re- word…resilience. Peter Levine suggests in *Trauma Proofing Your Kids* that resilience is the single most important gift we can foster in our children if we want them to be healthy.[2] I think he's right. Can we foster resilience in ourselves as well? Can we believe that whatever is coming at us could just as easily be a good thing as a bad one? Remember: "Don't sweat the small stuff: It's all small stuff." Do you recall the information about resetting the ventral vagus or social engagement system?

---

2   P. Levine (2008) *Trauma Proofing Your Kids*. Berkeley, CA: North Atlantic Books

Do you see the value of easing the pressure put on the entire bodymindcore with relaxation, movement, social engagement?

I'd argue most of us put our bodies into overdrive and never pay attention to what they're doing or how they feel. We hop out of bed, jump into the shower, get into our car or transport and land at our work space without ever stopping to check and ask our body "How do you feel today? What's working? What needs attention? What wants to be stretched to feel better?" We seem to have put our bodies on automatic pilot, ignoring signals that tell us we need to rest or slow down to feel these bodies. We choose instead to force posture and exert effort as we go through the day—being what we think the world wants us to be. It's like our body is a car with a "check engine" light blinking, and we've chosen to put tape over the warning light instead of having it serviced. If I could get all of us to consider one major idea, I think it would be this simple: **Slow down and listen to your body!** Communication with self is key to health.

Look at the Alternatives

I'd be remiss if I didn't mention looking at alternatives to the established medical route when you're in the preventative mode. Though my background is in bodywork and massage therapy, I've also explored and worked with nutritionists, acupuncturists, psychologists and counselors, biofeedback/ neurofeedback practitioners, chiropractors, osteopaths, craniosacral therapists, colonic therapists, energy healers, movement therapists, hypnotherapists, and so on. There are many good alternative practitioners out there who have different ideas about what can and should be done…to prevent a surgery, to prepare for one and to recover from it as well. Consider working with alternative ideas. Many doctors are great and want the best health outcomes for their patients, but most alternative practitioners got into their professions specifically to be helpful to others and without expectations of fame or fortune.

We notice in Dan's story he tried quite a few alternatives before giving in to surgery. He also had the luxury of a physical therapy background, so knew what he hoped to accomplish. Yet—he also gave us a very good warning when he invited us to realize that if we listen to our bodies, they will tell us they need rest, attention, movement, nutrition…but it's so easy to ignore these signals. Can you stop and look at self honestly, with common sense, and admit earlier in your process that *something* needs attention? Or will you, like too many of us, wait until it's too late to correct the difficulty and harsher measures are required?

And, as we explore alternatives, don't forget movement therapies! Whether you sign up for yoga classes, tai chi or chi gung, works with a Feldenkreis or Alexander or Laban movement specialist, visit the pool for water aerobics, attend dance classes or regular dances, pay to attend a fitness center or hire a personal trainer who takes you through a workout routine…always, keep moving! Remember my idea earlier in the book: If we pay someone to help us stay committed, chances are we'll work a bit harder to get our money's worth, and we'll also have a small desire to not let our guide down by missing our movement sessions.

I'd also be remiss if I didn't admit that some alternative practitioners feel a bit too ego-driven, believing in their "healing" powers. I always cringe when I see someone using the term "healer" to define their work. We, the practitioners, don't do the healing: A partnership led by our patron's inner knowing is necessary to elicit health; it's already within their being. So many practitioners believe in the power of their tool, and this is good. Yet no one tool or practitioner is right for everyone, just as every tool or practitioner is right for someone. Choose wisely when looking at alternatives (and doctors!) and trust your gut when you discuss a method with a practitioner partner. If it doesn't resonate for you, it's probably not going to be helpful.

Personally, I'd like to see us all, doctors and alternative folks, change the terminology around this healing relationship. I sometimes use the term "patron" to describe my clients…

patron denotes someone who seeks and appreciates my art. Likewise, I prefer the terms "practitioner partner" and "patron partner" when I think of this relationship.

And, while it's best to discuss with your doctor your work with an alternative practitioner, and the practitioner needs to know you're working with a doctor, remember, you are the captain and lead partner of your team! If your players can't or won't work together, something needs to change. A doctor who tells you to not work with someone, or a practitioner who tells you to only work with them, is suspicious to me right away! If everyone truly wants healing for you, do egos need to be involved? Or can we simply all work for the best good, together?

Often in this book we'll talk about social connectedness. Just as we know happily married people tend to live longer, studies show that clients who trust their practitioners continue to improve and feel better. Ask anyone who has a favorite massage therapist; they're often a large part of that person's support system. How many people really like and trust their doctors and look forward to visits? Happily, at least a few, and I believe these numbers are growing.

How to find the right practitioner for you? First, use your common sense and your gut wisdom. If you read about or discuss a treatment and think "That sounds really stupid/painful/worthless" you're probably right—for you. Ask yourself if this technique makes sense to you, in your head *and* your body. Does hearing and thinking about this idea tighten your body, or soothe it? Next look at the practitioner. Is this someone you feel you trust, as well as someone who both communicates well and makes you feel safe and cared for in your interactions? Do they seem to be demonstrating health and happiness to you? Why would you go to someone or try a technique that makes your guts tighter instead of more relaxed? Sometimes we're just not compatible. It's important to match your needs to a practitioner partner and a method that resonates for you.

There's nothing wrong with asking many questions when interviewing a practitioner. And there's nothing wrong with at least a phone call interview before you make a choice. If someone won't take the time to share their credentials, their model and their treatment plan, why would you want to invest your time in them and their work?

In a perfect world, each consumer of health care would be a wise and canny customer, asking the right questions and getting satisfactory answers before committing to working with a potential practitioner, allopathic or alternative. But this isn't that perfect world, and many of us need the guidelines that licensure and certification provide. It's important for you as consumer to scrutinize any relationship you'd consider forming with this person who may help you find your optimal health. Most good practitioners will welcome your questions and your desire to understand and participate in the treatment plan.

Do beware of authorities! I've known alternative practitioners I felt were abusers. If/when a client didn't improve under their guidance, the client would receive comments such as "You're just not trying hard enough" or "You must not want it enough." Again, not everyone can help every person in every situation…to believe it could be so is folly. When I discuss such a practitioner in my town with clients who *ask* my opinion, I often tell them some clients swear *by* that practitioner and others swear *at* him/her. I then invite them to go see the person, with an open mind but with a healthy dose of skepticism as well. I remember reading in the frontispiece of some book, many years ago, an "Admonition from the Buddha." It said something along the lines of "Beware of all proselytizing men; those who feel they have your answers…and beware of me also." I've always appreciated that sentiment.

All "healers" will have clients who resonate with them and all will have clients who don't; this truth doesn't make the practitioner or the clients "bad." None of us is right for everyone. I've often pondered about vibrations. As a musician, I think of vibration and harmony. Some people's keynote vibration of F# simply doesn't sound harmonious with my F! F# isn't a bad or wrong note; it just doesn't harmonize with my vibration. Any patron can and must discern, then decide what's harmoniously working for them with this practitioner partner with whom they resonate and feel positive results, *or not*.

Move It or Lose It: Using "That Which We Have"

If we're to prevent surgery, movement is critical! Remember my belief in the importance of movement, more often, where you are. *Any* activity can be an exercise, if we'll do it with a bit of awareness. I've decided we could all become healthier if we'd only practice *mindful movement*.

▌ If we're to prevent surgery, movement is critical!

Warning: Too many of us will faithfully work to prevent, or to prepare, or to recover. Then we'll begin to feel better, and we'll decide all is well, and fall off the wagon of self-care. We've all done this; good intentions turn into half-hearted attempts to keep up, into "I'll do that tomorrow—or the day after." Once you've decided to take charge of your process, it can be easy to let yourself off the hook and stop or slacken your workout routine. Therefore, begin small, slowly, taking a few steps instead of moving into a grand scheme, and finding you've failed or fallen by the wayside.

As I watch my 95-year-old father-in-law, I see him work hard to lift out of a chair. Sometimes he must lift/push up four or five times before developing the momentum to finally achieve an upright stance and move forward. But he doesn't stop trying! He continues to try until he rises again. And, as he lives alone in a two-story house with bathroom and bedroom on the second floor, he must stay active. I think it's prolonging his life to choose to live in such surroundings, moving as much as he can manage.

Pay Attention!

I'm reminded of the idea that maturity is the ability to discern finer and finer layers of distinction. I'd argue that maturity also allows us to slow down and examine more closely every aspect of what we're doing in our small personal universe. I remember a Rolf Movement instructor who had a skeletal issue and was told she wouldn't be able to walk if she overused her hip. She was still walking when I worked with her many years ago and told me at the time that she often spent *hours* making slow, deliberate, investigative self-movements that became smaller and smaller; more and more isolated and detailed in terms of finding and releasing tensions through the body. It's a talent I continue to emulate.

In movement or stillness, find *your* places. What hurts? Explore the pain, move, focus on it, stop and get to know it; move, focus above or below that sore place or make a slightly differently angled twist or roll or flexion or extension. Shift your body weight one way or another way. Observe what you can learn and how you can change the pain or discomfort. Once you feel that restricted place, stay. **Explore, breathe, move, feel. Take YOUR time! This slowed-down movement awareness work may be more important than any other work you find in your self-help quest.** When you've located a painful spot, take time to explore it. Perhaps you can roll over the spot on a tennis ball or foam roller. Perhaps putting your fingers or elbow into a spot and breathing into it can help you move congestion. Perhaps extending your body on a bench or leaning back in your chair to open the spine, or hanging from a doorway or putting your arms on a counter and lifting the upper body to "shake out" your spine will let you explore your stiffness and decide to change it.

Start somewhere! If you can only go three steps, celebrate those three, know you can do it, and plan on four tomorrow. If you can only lift yourself slightly out of an armchair, bless yourself and see what tomorrow or ten minutes brings as you sink back down into your chair. Praise yourself for the effort instead of cursing yourself for the failure. We're all in charge of our own process and responsible to motivate ourselves to change. Find the reasons you want to make positive changes and affirm that you're on track and change is coming. See it, feel it, visualize it, taste it, make it happen. And, remember, I know *my* process I've shared, based on my history…yours will be different. Follow it.

> Praise yourself for the effort instead of cursing yourself for the failure.

Much of what could fit into a "prevention" section of this book is already featured in the earlier part *Balance in All Things* and Chapter 6, *Mindful Movement, Where You Are*. If you skipped over those sections to get right to the "prevention" phase, I'd invite you to return and look more carefully at the ideas about bringing balance and movement into your life, as I believe that's the best prevention we can give ourselves. We can't necessarily heal ourselves from every trauma that may come to us, and we can't prevent every surgery in the world. But some simple attention to who we are and how we act, think and move can prolong our lives, postpone interventions and make us feel and live healthier. What do you have to lose?

LAST WORDS FROM THE DOCTOR

Noah quotes: "Our thoughts are prayers, and we are always praying." I would restate it slightly differently: We become what we focus on. If our day is filled with thoughts of chronic pain, or illness, or dysfunction, then our world is full of pain, dysfunction and usually without joy. **Chronic pain lives within our brain. People who focus on their pain often intensify and expand the scope of their pain.**

We say "Relax!" Too often I hear patients state: "Well, I try to relax." Perhaps Yoda said it best in *The Empire*

Strikes Back: "You must unlearn what you have learned. Try not. Do or do not. There is no try." Learning to relax to increase parasympathetic tone and self-regulation of our core body responses is not simple or easy, but profoundly important in health, healing and recovery.

There are two basic types of surgery: Emergency surgery, such as trauma from car accident or a hip fracture, or an acute illness such as an acute appendicitis; and elective surgery- something that is planned in advance. For both types, your overall health before surgery is profoundly important.

The medical community looks at test results, and images, but not necessarily at how people are functioning. In a study of middle-aged men who had never experienced back pain, 35 percent had a herniated disc, and over 55 percent had some kind of spinal abnormality—herniated disc, bulging disc, narrowing where the nerve comes out...but no pain.

Often, patients will describe themselves by their structural issues: "I have three herniated discs, and two bulging discs, and a bad knee," and "my neck has arthritis." But when I ask how often they are moving, or where they have joy or peace in their life, they have no answer. Life is defined by and restricted by their thinking, and their beliefs.

Face the Dragons Within

Whenever life makes me afraid
And I think nobody loves me, or I just want to die
I call the Master to make it right.
My burden is easy, and my yoke is light.

But I've got to face the dragons within;
I listen to their troubles and I give them my heart.
Once I have loved them they're free to depart,
But I've got to face the dragons within.

I've come into a strange new place…
A place I didn't know existed before.
I call the Master to see me through,
And what is before me to do, I do.

I just try to be the best I can be in the place that I am.
And when I die I hope that they'll say
I've done everything that I can.

But I've got to face the dragons within.
I listen to their troubles and I give them my heart.
Once I have loved them they're free to depart,
But I've got to face the dragons, we
should never kill the dragons!
I've got to face the dragons within.

Words and music by Noah Karrasch, from the
musical *Dear John: A New Revelation*

(based on the legend that Martha and Mary were exiled
from Jerusalem, washed up in France, and Martha
tamed a dragon after the crucifixion of Jesus)

8

Preparing for an Upcoming Surgery

DAN'S STORY

Finally, I came to the realization that I wasn't able to control my pain and I wasn't getting better. I made the decision to seek help. When I decided **something** had to change, I began asking around. Who had dealt with similar problems? What avenues did they explore, and how did they make their decisions? How satisfied with their decisions and treatments were they? There was so much information out there; one could be overwhelmed! The picture I drew from the information I acquired seemed like I'd be able to handle this trauma reasonably well.

Surgery requires anesthesia or a combination nerve block, which is a major traumatic event for anyone's body. Due to advances in most of the major surgeries such as bypass, joint replacement or spinal surgeries, to name a few, we've come to take for granted that such surgeries are relatively safe and simple procedures. However, all are traumatic to our bodies. Not only are we physically opened with a scalpel, but then bones are sawed off and replaced with artificial parts that must be essentially hammered into position to take the job of the removed parts. Any wonder why one is so very sore after a surgery? One must admit one's been badly treated, just as if one had been attacked and cut and beaten by someone on the street. Muscle and ligaments are pulled and stretched, and energy flow is disrupted by the cutting of muscles, nerves, blood vessels and connective tissue as well as the slowing effects of the drugs and anesthesia during and after the surgery. **Often little is done to prepare the individual for this traumatic event, or to plan on how the pain and energy disruption will be handled.**

I thought I'd prepared well; I'd asked around, I'd researched on the internet and talked to people with similar conditions about their treatments, and I'd studied the procedures and what I could expect. At the appointment with the orthopedic doctor I'd chosen to replace a hip gone bad, I asked what I thought were appropriate questions about the procedure, the time frame, the pain levels and most other questions that were in my mind.

Since I was a physical therapist and had worked with many of this physician's patients through the years, I witnessed first-hand that he always had great results. For years I'd heard from his patients that they didn't have post-op infections. Their surgical wound always healed well and their flexibility increased at a consistent rate which prevented later painful joint manipulation. This knowledge created a great sense of trust in this physician, so I decided to proceed rather than to seek out another surgeon about whom I knew little.

Keep Relaxing!

The first idea from *Prevention* bears repeating: Relax! You can focus on what could go wrong during or after surgery, and develop a worrisome, fear-based attitude, or like Dan you can choose to keep thoughts of failure out of the picture. Others have had a similar surgery before you; you can survive and thrive through yours as well. An attitude of gratitude instead of an attitude of fearfully proclaiming "Why me?" or "Whose fault is this? not mine!" can make everything go easier. Remember: "What you focus on expands." Or, reframed as Job said in the Bible: "That which I feared has come upon me." Did his thoughts attract those trials to him? Was he praying negatively by fearing what could go wrong?

Remember, whether you think you can or you can't, you're right. I think this applies to many aspects of life, including this goal of self-improved health, no matter where you sit on any medical spectrum or how intensive your treatment(s) may be. If you focus on the half empty picture of the glass, you'll worry, you'll find lack, you'll decide that problems could arise, and you'll think about them a lot. In doing so you'll magnify them and magnetize them to you. Research again shows how important attitude is in healing. How's your attitude? Remember, "our thoughts are prayers." Do you pray for pain by focusing on it?

On the other hand, you can focus on the positive thoughts: the people you know who've made it through similar challenges, the support team you have with you, the fact that you live in a place where help is available and your good fortune that professionals have the expertise to help you get better. Believe it, and you'll help to make it happen. Disbelieve, and you're inviting disaster. Don't worry about the next moment; just enjoy the present one.

Quantum physics realized some time ago that by simply observing an experiment, the observer becomes a part of that experiment, a participant. The outcome of an experiment is changed in part due to the expectations of that observer! If this is true, can't we change our own outcomes? Can't we magnetize and/or hypnotize ourselves to expect an outcome that brings positive energy to us instead of negative? Or do we *prefer* the worry, partly because it makes us *feel* something? Years ago, I created an acronym for worry: Worthless Old Rotten Recycled Yuck. Why recycle the yuck instead of looking for the good?

If it's true that "what we focus on expands," why not spend time talking to your body? Bless it, thank it for the good it's doing. Encourage it to respond, to perform, to heal. Listen! Have a conversation with your body; find out what it wants from you. Many of us have realized if we talk to our cells and tissues to prepare for surgery, the recovery may be much smoother. A bit of mental preparation, lowering the anxiety and believing the body wants to heal; these things can make recovery so much better. Recall how Dan went into surgery knowing recuperation would be difficult, but that others had already accomplished that healing and he could do so as well. While you're special and unique, you're not your doctor's first rodeo!

> You can focus on the positive thoughts... Believe it, and you'll help to make it happen. Disbelieve, and you're inviting disaster. Don't worry about the next moment; just enjoy the present one.

Choosing Your Team: Supportive Connections

Talk to your doctors to get the answers you need. If you can't get answers from a doctor, keep trying, and, if necessary, find another doctor. Ask the hard questions: You and your questions are important, and unasked questions simply fester and leave seeds for worries to grow. Don't try to create problems, but be realistic that problems can occur, and find out what those problems might be so you can minimize them in your own head and even avoid them.

> **QUESTIONS FOR YOUR DOCTOR**
> - What is the procedure?
> - What are its goals?
> - What are the risks?
> - Are you using current technology, or are you doing things the way you've always done them?
> - What has changed? Why aren't you changing as well?
> - What is the ballpark figure of time in surgery?

- How long will I be in hospital? How long does healing take?
- What tasks can I perform at what time points?
- What can go wrong, and how often does that happen?
- What are my chances of making a complete recovery?
- What's a good guess of the costs financially to me?
- Is there anything else I should be/might be asking you that would be helpful to me?

The last is a question I often ask when I'm in information-gathering mode, whether in a medical setting or any place I want to garner more ideas before I decide. This invitation to your practitioner partner can often bring ideas and information you hadn't even thought about. After I've exhausted my questions, and my authority, I usually end by asking some form of this question. What do you have to lose, and what do you have to gain by asking?

In addition to talking with your doctors and other medical staff, make sure you have a support system of at least one listening ear from a friend or family member. **Find someone who will listen, offer support and a bit of stern talk if/when you need and as you can accept it from them.** Know what you want from them, let them know what you need, and you'll have a better relationship. I'm lucky to have a family member who's a family practice doctor. If or when I can't get answers or clarifications, I call him for help and consultation. Even without your personal physician you can solicit help and ideas from friends and even strangers on the internet. Most surgeries and conditions have chat groups full of people who have already lived your fears. Get connected, somehow.

For years, whenever my partner Gloria would "complain" to me about a situation, I'd jump right into "fix-it" mode, trying to offer advice or a direction she might want to consider following to "solve" the problem. Quite often, I'd get an edgy

"I don't want advice; I just want you to listen." This was when I learned it's helpful to set the rules for what you want from such a relationship. Do you want someone who will nudge you when they see you falling into negativity? Or do you just want sympathy and cookies? Both are appropriate, and both may come from the same friend…but your friend needs and wants to know what you expect from them—in any moment— if they're to be your best sounding board. The clearer your communications about your needs, the better your chances will be to get those needs met.

Most of us, facing surgery, have fears. This is normal. Finding others to validate our right to fears, while helping us face them, can be an important part of healing. Fear is an obstacle that must be broken down if we're to understand exactly what our individual fear is about. As with any stressors, how we perceive our fears and to what degree we allow them to pervade our world will direct our thoughts, actions, and ultimately our healing. I remember years ago seeing a book title: *Feel the Fear and Do It Anyway*.[1] This seems like the appropriate response to fear— own it, process it, move through it. I repeat my current mantra around my fears: Find it, face it, feel it, forget it. Hopefully you'll find support on your way through the fear…don't be afraid to ask! Do you see we're back to facing our problems, to "feeling" instead of fighting, fleeing or freezing?

Information Gathering

Talking to friends and family can be helpful but also confusing, as so many people have stories, both good and bad, about exactly what you're considering. Likewise, internet searches can be helpful…chances are, you'll find reviews from people who tell you the procedure you're having is the best thing that ever happened to them. Others will swear it's the worst. Both are correct; it's only in our personal event that we truly learn, and

1   S. Jeffers (1987) *Feel the Fear and Do It Anyway*. New York, NY: MJF Books.

your personal event is coming. Thus, none of these people or sites can give you your best information, but, taken together, they can give you a lot of information and help you understand the procedure, the risks, the rewards and the challenges other people have experienced. Gathering information is not a bad thing.

I've heard that many doctors wish patients wouldn't go to the internet, getting ideas in their head about what's going on, what might happen, because patients often self-diagnose and misdiagnose their condition. I can understand that attitude from a doctor. I can also understand that a caring doctor appreciates a patient who works to try to understand their situation better to be prepared for the future and its eventualities. If your doctor isn't on board with your seeking information, is s/he a caring caregiver?

Talking to others who know something about the surgery you're considering, or committing to, can also be helpful. You're not the first to go through this situation, so check with friends and relatives and listen to their stories. Your surgeon should be able to provide a couple of names of patients who have successfully completed the same or similar procedures. Remember Dan had the luxury of seeing many patients who had worked with the doctor he chose over his years in a physical therapy career. It was easy for him to make his decision based on their input and his desire to avoid infection after the surgery. For most of us it's a bit more complex to negotiate the choices. You don't have to become wedded to someone else's story and assume it will go the way it's gone for them, but the more information you can gather, the less surprises you'll have in the long run. Once information is collected, how we sort it to use it also is important.

I've already mentioned most of us do well to have an "advocate" when we visit our doctor…someone who can help us clarify both the questions we want to ask and the answers we're receiving. We all know doctors are busy folks who are often on a tight schedule. Most doctors truly don't have time to stay around and answer questions, much less visit.

The more you can write out and prioritize your questions, then bring your advocate to help you get and understand answers, the more satisfied you'll be with doctor visits. I remember my surgeon from those plane wreck days; he'd waltz into the room, answer one question and try to get away. I'd have my list of questions for him, with my partner there to help get answers. Usually he'd be backing out of the room by question two. Not a helpful healer!

> I've already mentioned most of us do well to have an "advocate" when we visit our doctor...someone who can help you clarify both the questions you want to ask and the answers you're receiving.

AnesthesiAnathema

I paired the two words above because your anesthesia can be your anathema! While it's great to not be made aware of the pain and trauma your body goes through when you're in surgery, it's also good to be made aware of the possible side effects of the drugs introduced into your system to keep you relaxed and pain free while surgery progresses. A bit of foreknowledge about both what you can do beforehand and what you may expect after is useful in preparing yourself for that which is to come.

First, your doctor and anesthetist need to know about all the medications you're taking...but, also, about your vitamin regimen, your herbal regimen, your alcohol, tobacco and drug regimen, especially opiates and cocaine! This isn't the time to hide behaviors; that little white lie could get you into a world of problems if you choose to pretend you're drug- and alcohol-free. If you are preparing for surgery, it's best to cut out as much consumption as you can...in the long run, the cleaner you are, the better your chance of having fewer problems. While, statistically, only about one person in a quarter of a million dies as a result of anesthesia during or after surgery (and others do have reactions), why not be as prepared as possible? Your medical history is important, and a large part of that history, beyond conditions, is consumptions. So be honest with yourself and your doctors.

Do you have allergies? Some of us are allergic to drugs introduced commonly into the body during surgery. Perhaps you've not yet experienced a surgery, so don't know. But if you're aware of any problems with surgical drugs in the past, make sure your anesthesiologist knows.

Generally, drugs are induced into your body to both relax you and to take away the pain. Usually either through inhalation or through needles, the drugs are brought into you. Fairly soon you'll be sleepy, loopy and float away…usually while you're counting backward or some such procedure to let your anesthetist know you're actually "going out." Don't fight, just allow. The anesthetic will suppress the autonomic system as well as stifle pain, so your breath, circulation, heart rate, digestive system and swallowing mechanism may all be compromised. This is why you'll often have a tube placed down your throat while you're "under." This tube allows you to breathe deeply when your systems are cutting back on the work they do.

But, be aware, this throat tube can cause injury or irritate the throat and the larynx as well! You may wake up with coughing, sore throat, hoarseness and a gag reflex. My gag reflex from the last surgery was particularly severe…for many days, every time I tried to brush my teeth, I nearly vomited. Just the simple act of sticking the toothbrush in my mouth—not even deeply— caused me to gag violently. In fact, seven days after surgery, on my discharge day, while brushing my teeth I reacted so violently that I had to grab the sink basin and hold on for dear life for several minutes before I regained equilibrium.

Once you're out of recovery, other problems may occur. Some happen fairly often and aren't as serious; for example, it's common to have nausea and vomiting. You may also experience headaches and tiredness, especially for the first several days, possibly even a couple of weeks. You may shiver or tremble; you may feel confused and disoriented. Personally, I believe some longer-term mental confusion comes from receiving anesthesia as well. Without research, I'd suggest that for me, it took much longer than two weeks for my brains to feel they were totally with me; I'd say it was more like several months before I mentally felt myself again.

Other, more serious effects can occur, leading up to that *very* rare death: Blood pressure and heart rate can increase dramatically. Allergic reactions, *infections*, lung problems, high fever and irritation from both throat tube and IV needle sticks can cause pain in the throat or the muscle tissue where the stick occurred. Most seriously but *very* occasionally, heart and stroke issues can be caused by receiving drugs during surgery.

So, while most of us want to be "out" for that surgery, it's best to be prepared by keeping yourself as clean as possible before the surgery, sharing with your doctor the truth about your consumption habits and knowing that after surgery you won't be "right" for a length of time. Don't force yourself to come back from this trauma until your body is ready! Take your time, realize you may be unbalanced for as much as a couple of weeks, or more, and allow the process to work. You'll sort it out after, if you're prepared before your time.

Learn from My Mistakes: Protection

I made some mistakes with my recent two surgeries. The first surgery for that perforated colon felt necessary to me. For 29 years I'd managed to keep functioning, but I could tell I was having more difficulty with bowel movements. The sigmoid colon was removed; I was left with a hole in my abdomen through which to empty my bowel and poor instruction as to what to do with this new life. As the situation was identified to me as critical and emergency, I listened; then gave permission for the first surgery. I had no time to prepare! I was shocked, but hoped I was doing the right thing…in fact, I couldn't see any alternatives. I made peace and did what I could to rehabilitate myself, with little second-guessing as to whether I'd done the right thing. And frankly, I did "sail through" (not without pain, but with fast forward progress).

The second and more recent surgery was another matter, however. I thought I'd sought out the correct information and questions. I met Dr. One (he who had examined me on the first emergency visit and discussed with me but didn't perform the first surgery) a month before the surgery date we chose for reconstruction, to discuss the pros and cons. I'd already done some research and thought I knew what the procedure would entail. I had my list of questions ready for the visit. Sadly, I wish I'd thought of a few more questions.

Let me detour by saying I had had "gut" reactions to this surgeon, Dr. One, from that first painful morning when he talked to me in the emergency room, telling me what procedure was planned but letting me know he was too busy so was turning me over to an associate. I told him that for years I'd worked to keep the bowels clear because when too much pressure from my gut pushed on my bladder, I had issues with bladder incontinence. He basically told me I was being ridiculous because the bowel and bladder had no relationship whatsoever. My gut clenched at his disdain for common sense. After that invalidation, I thought "I don't want to work with this man." Remember I earlier suggested you trust your gut around your helper team? This, I did not do.

When a few hours later I met his associate, Dr. Two, who was to do the emergency colostomy, immediately I was reassured by his demeanor, his attitude, his caring. I asked him after a short visit: "Would you also take on the reconstruction surgery when the time comes?" He assured me Dr. One was far better equipped to handle the second, more complicated surgery. I still had doubts, until I spoke with a nurse whom I trusted above all I saw during my five days of that first hospitalization. She reassured me that though Dr. One was "no warm fuzzy," technically he was brilliant and that if she needed such a surgery she'd want him to do it. I was swayed, even though every time I met and talked with this doctor, alarm bells rang in my head. Nevertheless, I stayed with him and allowed him to do this second procedure. My choice.

So, in our visit to discuss the second procedure, he answered my questions and we scheduled the surgery. He assured me that, as the first surgery had gone well, we could expect the same thing from the second. Where I'd spent five days in hospital with the first surgery, he told me I'd very probably be released in three to five days. He mentioned my scar would be a tiny bit longer, reiterating that there were no guarantees as to the positive outcome of my bowels working more fully, but that, overall, it was likely this would be something a bit more strenuous than a walk in the park. I left with the impression that I'd sail through this surgery since I'd rehabilitated very well from the first. I thought I'd done things correctly, so I'd have a fairly easy time with this surgery and recovery.

Well, on recovering, the pain was far more severe; the scar had grown by about an additional 60 percent, from six inches to ten. My spleen felt totally violated and bruised from the procedure of pulling the colon off the spleen to reconnect the shortened colon with its descending colon. To add insult to injury, even though I planned to take probiotics while in hospital, the doctor forbade it…"nothing by mouth"—except for the pills he wanted me to take, but no probiotics, which I saw as critical to staying healthy.

Sure enough, on day three I was diagnosed with *Clostridium difficile*. The bacteria *C. diff* produces highly contagious spores which are spread through feces. When one who is exposed to these spores (which are becoming rampant in many hospitals and nursing homes) and has taken strong antibiotics, those drugs kill most of the bad bacteria. For some reason *C. diff* thrives in antibiotics. It becomes stronger, causing diarrhea (mine lasted 60 hours!) and incredible weakness. Besides that, I became a pariah—isolation, double gowns and gloves, no visitors. And, once the spores have invaded your body, according to current medical science they'll be with you always, and you're four times as likely to have a recurrence. My best "medical" advice: Take probiotics! Yet this doctor wouldn't let me take them before the *C. diff* occurred, and I allowed him to be my authority. I felt betrayed, by him and by myself.

Other signals kept telling me I'd chosen my team poorly; assurances that I'd be able to work and travel at three weeks because I'd done so after the first surgery proved false. Dr. One forced me to try to urinate on my own even though I'd urinated primarily through stomach muscles for nearly 30 years, and those muscles were now cut, compromised and hurting. The urologist I subsequently saw immediately insisted I temporarily use catheters instead of pushing with those damaged stomach muscles. Nearly every bit of advice I got from Dr. One ended up feeling like it contributed more to my problems. Finally, I decided Dr. One's work was about him and his world, not mine. Technically he was a good doctor, but he honored his needs, not mine.

The second surgery's scar is a work of art! It's healed reasonably well and much of the pain was gone seven weeks after surgery. However, many months after surgery, inside my stomach I still felt bruised and damaged. By not listening to my gut, and not looking outside the medical network of care my insurer provided, I think I went through more pain than was necessary. Heed my tale of woe; talk to your doctor or doctors to get the answers and reassurances you need before you say "yes" to their recommendations.

After this second recent surgery, I've since talked to quite a few people who have an example of how the "takedown" surgery to repair and reconnect is far worse than that first colostomy surgery. Yet Dr. One insisted it would go well, even easily, so I didn't ask about a patient I might visit about my questions. In hindsight, I wish I'd sought more opinions from others who had gone through the procedure *before* making my decision.

Back to Basic Fuels: Probiotics and Other Precautions

Let's return to probiotics: I highly recommend them; not only before the surgery but after as well. Whether your doctor says yes or no, probiotics make common sense. If, during surgery, one takes *anti*biotics, to kill all the bad stuff, what's happened to the good stuff? It's been killed as well! That's why *probiotics* make so much sense. And while good yogurts (not the fruit/sugar varieties) also make sense, probiotic capsules are far more convenient. A traveling nurse I met told me of a hospital in Virginia where she'd worked in orthopedic surgery. Doctors there had experimented and found that prescribing and using probiotic doses before *and* after orthopedic surgery gained their patients much quicker healing time.

Generally, probiotics are very good for treating diarrhea, enhancing the immune system and possibly enhancing protection against allergies as well, but this new use to prepare for surgery and enhance recovery and to continue their use after is exciting. Dr. One said no to probiotics and I still wonder... could I have prevented *C. diff*? My regular doctor had gotten me on probiotics immediately after the first colon surgery and advised me to stay with them...which I happily did, until Dr. One told me they weren't part of the treatment plan. My plan, yes; his plan, no. Why did I give away my power?

I'd suggest trying a probiotic for about four weeks to see if you like the effects before any upcoming surgery. If a surgery comes on you by surprise, get probiotics into your system as quickly as you can to alleviate the antibiotic's killing effect on your good bacteria. Chances are you'll feel your digestion and elimination is smoother; you may experience symptoms such as diarrhea or breaking out. If so, try another probiotic. There are many on the market. Also, if you begin taking them, you'll want to stay with them at least through the surgery and recovery time. They can't last in the system; they will run through it. You must continue taking them to benefit and restore your good gut bacteria, and especially while you're taking or have recently taken antibiotics.

Interestingly, I'd been using a specific probiotic faithfully since the first colon surgery and planned to continue in the hospital until the doctor "forbade" their use. A nutritionist friend has since told me this specific probiotic can kill *C. diff*! I do wish I'd listened to my gut, which was crying for any probiotic during the last hospital visit.

Three categories of medicine/supplement are meant to help us stay clean on the inside: antibiotics, probiotics and prebiotics. Each is named appropriately: Antibiotics kill off life and get rid of pathogens which make us sick, probiotics add to life and prebiotics are meant to help one maintain a healthy gut environment. Antibiotics have been used far too indiscriminately over the past 50 years, with the result that the bacteria meant to be controlled have evolved into new forms that are able to combat many of our current antibiotics. This is the simplest reason that using antibiotics sparingly makes sense...especially as many of us use them for colds and other viral infections over which they have no power whatsoever, while they kill both good and bad bacteria in our systems.

Antibiotics work in three ways: either they shoot holes into bacteria, poison them or destroy their ability to reproduce. But they have no effect on viruses, and can be particularly hard for children and old people who are less stable and less able to recover after treatments. It's common sense to keep them as a top shelf remedy instead of a default mechanism whenever we have a slight problem. While they will kill most bacteria, there will always be others that manage to remain, survive and thrive. It's good advice to take antibiotics sparingly (unless they're really necessary), and instead to buy organic, to wash fruits and vegetables carefully, to wash your hands more often and to be aware that when traveling abroad you'll probably ingest new bacteria. If you follow these simple rules chances are you may not need antibiotics as often as you think you do.

> Antibiotics work in three ways: either they shoot holes into bacteria, poison them or destroy their ability to reproduce. But as they have no effect on viruses, and as they can be particularly hard for children and old people... it's common sense that we should keep them as a top shelf remedy instead of a default mechanism whenever we have a slight problem.

Most people don't talk about prebiotics at all; you might choose to call this type of medicine "fiber" or "roughage." Prebiotics are simply those foods that truly help you because they feed the good bacteria in your system. Obviously fresh fruits and many vegetables are among the best foods: what I think of as "roots and fruits" in the "medicines" section of my foods chart (Table 3.1 in Chapter 3). If you see all root vegetables as healthy foods, plus any vegetables that have seeds inside the "fruit," you're eating healthier, prebiotic foods. Garlic, onions, leeks, parsnips, turnips, beets, carrots, potatoes and sweet potatoes are among the healthy roots. Tomatoes, green beans, zucchini and other squash, peppers, peas and okra are among the healthier "fruit" vegetables with seeds inside. Spinach and other greens, cabbage, broccoli and cauliflower, those vegetables without seeds inside, are actually best eaten cooked instead of raw, in terms of altering their chemistry to make them more digestible.

Most of us believe whole grains are better for us than highly processed flours, but currently much of what I believe is labelled gluten intolerance may be simply the body's response to the poisonous glyphosate added to our grains to make them grow resistant to insects. Healthier foods tend to be prebiotic. You can also find prebiotic supplements at a pharmacy or health food store when you're ready to feed your bacteria good foods. As good bacteria are good for us, why shouldn't we feed them health foods as well?

I was amazed in my last hospital visit when, knowing I had *C. diff* and wanting to try to heal that condition by adding good stuff to my system, I ordered yogurt. The kitchen staff person who took my order obviously felt I wasn't eating enough...she sent yogurt, *and* jello, *and* apple juice, *and* ice cream! When I looked at the ingredients and realized all were full of sugar, I ate very little. Why add fuel that fuels the sickness?

In general, hospital nutritionists have a different idea of healthy eating than I do. When ordering, I specified I didn't want a suggested item because of sugar content. The immediate response was, "Oh, we have sugar-free!" No, thank you. I personally believe that as time goes on, more and more research will show that artificial sweeteners are truly causing more harm to our systems than doing good. And do we really need six different kinds of potatoes on the menu, with five of them some form of fried food? Do we need so much white flour in our diets, especially when the flour has been made from treated grains? Do all the meats need to be breaded and fried, or cooked into oblivion? Perhaps this is what patients want, but, if healthier choices were presented, wouldn't patients eat better foods instead? Remember our chart of nutritious foods versus poisons? With which part of that chart do you primarily relate?

And let me reiterate: I'm not a nutritionist, I only share common sense. The fresher, least processed foods tend to be the healthiest foods. If you're only eating dried and processed foods from packages, or fast foods from drive-in "restaurants," chances are you're poisoning yourself. The more you search out foods you can enjoy which have health values, the happier your body will be.

Cleanliness Is Next to Godliness: What Are We Inhaling or Touching?

Hospital precautions are only as good as the staff's habits, and too often the staff are overworked. It's easy to make small mistakes; perhaps because they're on 12-hour shifts, but simple sloppiness or laziness will cause mistakes to happen. You may have heard the statistic that physician and hospital errors are now the third leading cause of death in the USA. Between missed diagnoses, medical mistakes and airborne or touch-borne germs, hospitals are a great place to get sick, but often not such a good place to *be* sick.

I remember visiting a 90-year-old friend in hospital several years past. She'd fallen and broken her wrist and hip and had been through horrible surgeries to repair them. Lying in the bed, she was crying and thrashing. A housekeeper very kindly wanted to comfort her. I watched the woman put down her mop, take off her gloves, then move the dirty mop handle with bare hands before taking the hands of the patient. Truthfully, I didn't stop the housekeeper, because the deed was already done when I realized what I'd seen, and a 90-year-old with Alzheimer's may be ready to depart. I didn't see any ability to change the outcome of what had just happened. I was a bad advocate.

In my own last hospital stay, I witnessed a nurse drop something on the floor as she was preparing my pills and injection. As I couldn't yet turn to see what happened, I didn't know what it was. I do know it fell right on the floor in an area where I'd leaned over the bed and vomited hours earlier, that had never been totally cleaned! At this stage I was in so much pain that by the time I'd worked into my mental process what had just happened, we were past the incident and the drugs were already in my system, possibly compromised. Was that my intro to *C. diff*? Possibly. Don't be afraid or ashamed to confront staff when you see them violating universal precautions. It could save your life. And, remember, having a second set of eyes is helpful! Where's that advocate?

Another thought: Usually you see the staff wash hands frequently, sometimes both before and after dealing with the patient in hospital. How often do you see a patient's hands being washed? You might add Clorox wipes, or at least antibacterial wipes, to your kit of equipment to take to your hospital visit. Let's remember that we can add precautions even when the staff slip up on theirs.

Another condition to be avoided, a large problem in hospitals, is sepsis or blood infection. Sepsis happens when the body responds to an infection and begins to injure its own tissues and organs. It comes when an immune response triggers the infection, commonly from a bacterium, but it could also come from a virus, fungus or parasite. Antibiotics and intravenous fluids are usually the treatment course. As this is a leading cause of death, we again want to do all that's possible to remain clean, healthy and germ-free while in the hospital, and at home afterwards, as well.

And yet one more difficult hospital problem is MRSA, or methicillin-resistant *Staphylococcus aureus*. MRSA is a bacterium, now quite common in hospitals, nursing homes and prisons. Without treatment, this can be another deadly problem. Yet, simple precautions often help; for example, placing iodine around the nose of the patient, before the surgery, to prevent accepting the bacterium into the system. Again, precautions, before and after surgery! Be in charge, not only of your body, but the way others treat it. A bit of tea tree oil around your nose, placed by you, may have the same effect as iodine. Listen to the man who wasn't as thorough as he might have been! Be vigilant when you get to the hospital; prepare yourself to be watchful towards staff violations of cleanliness and common sense.

More than 95 percent of the bacteria in the world are harmless to humans, and many of us have many of them in our systems, without problems. Many are extremely beneficial. If we'll remember to handle our foods with cleanliness and common sense we usually can keep the "bad ones" at bay.

One item I pack in my travel kit in pretty much all my travels (and didn't use as well as I should have on this last surgery, thus possibly helping me contract *C. diff*) is tea tree oil. Years ago I met a chiropractor who'd walked across much of Australia with Aborigines. She spoke of that culture's use of tea tree oil, also called melaleuca. I started using it as well. I've been known to even brush my teeth with it if I have no toothpaste, and any scratch or open sore usually gets a dose of tea tree oil.

In the USA, when we clean we tend to get rid of and kill everything as we achieve cleanliness, and I'm convinced this isn't such a good idea. Studies have shown that children with two or more pets have far fewer allergies than their peers who have one or no pets. The "new and improved" antibacterial soaps that kill everything frankly kill so many pathogens that germs are evolving in ways that make the new and improved product ineffective. We don't need to clean so obsessively; in many countries with lower cleaning standards there are far lower incidences of allergies and autoimmune diseases.

Cleaning doesn't mean killing all bacteria, but suggests we find a healthy balance of enough good bacteria with a few bad ones and stay in that healthy balance. New research has even suggested washing in hot water is actually no more effective than thorough washing in cold water!

The Root of All Evil?

Let's talk about money. First, let me say I can't solve all your problems, though I wish I could. I wish to give you ideas and hope, little else. We all know medical care can be tremendously expensive; in part because of the prescription of tests that rule out conditions that might manifest, but also because of malpractice insurance rates, and lawsuits that come when someone's lawyer feels their doctor hasn't been thorough. We also know Big Pharma makes a great deal of money, more in this country than in most others...they're certainly getting good return on their investments of developing drugs! Add to this the idea that drug reps visit doctors, bring free lunches and other *stuff,* and convince the clinic to try this "new and improved" brand of treatment...it's a sick system, our medical care! And participating in it takes a lot of money, especially if your insurance program isn't that good or your finances aren't perfectly sound—and even if they are.

Years ago a client came to me. She'd been doing quite well with a heart condition on her medical regimen, until her doctor had a visit from a drug representative who brought a "new and improved" medicine, which the doctor then prescribed for my client. Shortly after taking this new medication, the woman's lungs filled with fluid and she required open heart surgery. She never recovered from that insult, and her husband never let go of the idea that if she hadn't been switched from what was working and onto the "new and improved" he'd still have her with him. But the young drug rep made a nice sale, and the doctor had another nice lunch served to his staff. Money really does seem to be the root of much evil, if not all.

How can one get better if one is focused on the lack of money? If I'm lying awake at night worrying about bills, how can I feel better in the morning after a poor sleep? It's sad but true; it's easy to get focused on the lack of money around medical care, but it's most important to focus on healing and affirm that, somehow, the money will be dealt with after the healing has taken place. Too many of us are in a tough position in this regard. Health care is already expensive and that anxiety over money can certainly make us sicker.

Can you let it go? As you prepare for a surgery, can you allow yourself to let the money worries go as well? Can you do what it takes to get as well as you can, and allow money to sort itself after the fact?

> How can one get better if one is focused on the lack of money? If I'm lying awake at night worrying about bills, how can I feel better in the morning after a poor sleep?

Perhaps there will be financial challenges or a bankruptcy in your future based on your insurance coverage or lack thereof and your ability to pay off medical debts, but **it's the present you must focus your energy toward** if you're going to be able to get well.

A neighbor told me recently that his world was fine until he was prescribed a new medication; immediately he developed blood clots in his leg and fears he may lose it. A client tells me his new medication swelled his legs; though he's now off that med, the legs are taking a long time to release the effects. These stories and others make me leery of overmedications. When medicine is appropriate, I'll take it; but I'm going to be very discerning as to how much medicine I'll take. On this last hospital visit I only used painkillers for three days...yes, I hurt, but I wanted that stuff out of my system, thinking both of potential liver damage and of the ability of such drugs to slow down the digestive and eliminative systems.

One of the few "medications" I have no objection to people using is sleep aids. Common sense tells us if we can't get restful sleep it's harder to heal. I'm fine with using whatever sleep aids I can find to reclaim good rest. I've had clients tell me they're so happy to hear an "alternative" practitioner tell them sleep aids may be a good thing for them…sometimes, alternative folks shun any such help. I say, get your sleep, first! Hopefully you won't get addicted to sleep aids, but, in the short term, restful sleep is critical.

Several years ago I attended an integrative medicine conference where the physician keynote speaker told of a 95-year-old patient brought in by his daughters. He was on 25 different medications! As the doctor was able to wean the man off ALL the meds, he became amazingly healthy! I often wonder just how much of this overmedication is going on in our world. And think of the costs! Someone profited handsomely from this older gent's use of medications; it wasn't him.

Make no mistake: We're focused on the business of *health* care, which could more appropriately be called "*sick* care." There's little health in much of what is done to patients. And too much is done to make money for someone. It's frustrating to be a patient, know your dollars must be stretched, and be forced into using expensive medications which may or may not be doing your body any good. I've recently thought, more and more, how alternative practitioners try to restore energetic movement, and medical practitioners too often try to stop or slow it.

With the high cost of "health" care only increasing, if money is an issue that's causing concern, exploring options might bear some fruit and give the team a feeling of doing *something*: Is there a generic version of the drug you need that's less expensive but as effective? Is there some alternative you might use? Is surgery absolutely necessary, or somewhat elective? Do you know the success rate of the proposed surgery? Would or could you try an alternative treatment? Have you made friends with your pharmacist, who often knows much more about drugs than your physician? How much will your insurance cover in each choice? Could you consider "medical tourism" to a country where you can afford the surgery for less money? Does the drug manufacturer have any kind of charity program to help you cover expenses? Often, there are subsidies or help available, if we only knew where to look. Sometimes your doctor can give you samples from the drug reps to save you money. Discuss your concerns with your doctor, before surgery if possible, and see if s/he has options you hadn't considered. Shop among the pharmacies; prices can vary widely between shops. Explore options!

It's also difficult to focus on healing if you do have insurance but must fight with your insurer, who doesn't want to cover a condition for whichever of many reasons they might find or invent. It's hard to believe in the caring of *any* insurance executives when their yearly salaries and "bonuses" for their hard work are astronomical. I'll step off my soap box soon, but not before I say that there will probably be some sort of karmic justice for those who prey on the less fortunate to enhance their own fortunes. And there seems to be a great deal of this form of preying in our world today. It can make you sick!

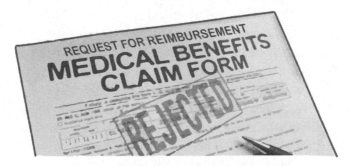

Sadly, too much of medicine is about "bottom line"
and saving the insurance company money.

Most countries have some sort of health care system offering treatment to their citizens whether they have the money or insurance resources to pay or don't. The USA is still behind on this front. Yes, everyone can get treatment in an emergency room situation, but that's another reason medical costs have skyrocketed. In every country medical care has its problems, but only in the USA are we totally without compassionate basic care available to all regardless of financial ability. Many Americans declare bankruptcy yearly, and too many of these bankruptcies are medically induced. A civilized society can and should do better.

Meanwhile, in the here and now, in nearly any community or family the lack of money can be a tremendous burden. Remembering to develop that attitude of gratitude will often help one overcome the fear of lack that prevails when one begins to consider the costs of medical treatments. Focusing on small victories while keeping worry over money at bay can help you heal; focusing on how destitute you've become won't help you feel better! It's tough to admit, but true. Whether you can afford treatments or not, if they keep you alive, chances are you'll want to take treatments and worry later. If at all possible, put that worry off until later, when you are better equipped to deal with it.

And Again, You Are How You Move: Motivation

And a final important preparation to help your body be at its best condition for the coming insult: still, and always, move more. Everything discussed in the first section about prevention still makes sense. Whatever movements you choose to make, make them! Don't just think about them, wish they were done, then forget them. Walk! Stretch! Flex, twist and bend/extend. If truly we all suffer from motion starvation, realize you may have been starving your body more than is possibly healthy (or you probably wouldn't be facing many of the surgeries most of us are now facing). Start moving that machine. Even if it's hard to get out of the chair, lift yourself with your arms, as far as you can lift, several times in a row. Sit and move your feet; toes up, down, heels up, down. Draw circles with your feet. If that's all you can do, do it, keep trying to do it and, hopefully, get a bit better at it. Don't beat yourself up if you can't move well; just keep exploring how to add more movement to your life.

Interestingly, there have been studies showing that simply visualizing movement has benefit. Even if you're stuck in your chair, or your bed, can you "see" yourself moving, walking, exercising? Using such visualization may well get you started physically moving, much quicker.

But if you can move well enough, why aren't you walking? For some time I've used walking as part of my prevention, preparation and rehabilitation. I can't think of anything quite as valuable as just getting a decent walk every day or every other day. And I've realized that if I'll walk with my head up and waist held back it seems to activate the core of my body in a way that I feel I get a far better workout. Try it—paying attention to the way you hold your body as you walk, see if you can develop a better walking posture.

So, I've suggested a great deal of preparation of the physical variety…take the step towards movement, whatever those steps can be for you. Perhaps just pushing yourself out of bed twice a day is all you can accomplish. Do it. Perhaps you know taking a walk is important but just can't make time for it. Make it. Perhaps you'd like to take a yoga class but are reluctant to pay the fees when you're not sure you'll stay with it. Pay it and stay with it. We could all be doing more to prepare ourselves; most of that preparation could also be prevention if we'll only start early enough in our quest to be healthier. Once you know a surgery is coming, why *not* double down on common sense ideas that will help you move through your surgery without complications?

Much of what I'm suggesting in this preparation for surgery section continues to be important after the surgery as well… why add sugar to the diet when you're trying to heal? Why allow someone to examine you if they won't meet your standards of cleanliness? Why not wash your hands more frequently instead of less frequently? Why aren't you moving more and eating healthier foods? In lesser quantities?

You may want a "packing list" for your hospital stay: I take tea tree oil, cranberry concentrate, probiotics and Clorox wipes, in addition to books, puzzles and things to keep me entertained.

You might even consider earplugs, though they may only frustrate you a bit more.

Preparation for that upcoming surgery can make things go so much better! Remember, first prepare your mental attitude and then take the steps: Move, eat well, clear your fear thoughts, research what's going to happen, get clear with your doctor. In all ways, clean yourself out from the negativity; the bad foods, the bad thoughts, the lack of movement, the lack of proper hygiene habits. The better prepared you are, the better your chances of a successful outcome when you do surrender to the drugs and the procedure.

LAST WORDS FROM THE DOCTOR

Hospitals are not places of health. A patient's day and night will seem chaotic; nothing is familiar and the patient has very little control over themselves. Noah states: "You can focus on the positive thoughts." This is profoundly true. It is very easy for patients to focus only on the negative, or the unknown. Too often, patients don't ask questions, so the unknowns and the fears run uncontrolled. Regarding fear and "Find it, face it, feel it, forget it...," I would add: Name IT! The ability to name a situation or process is the beginning of resolution.

Have an Advocate! The medical model is often based upon: "The doctor talks, the patient listens and accepts." Good health requires conversation and understanding. The patient who is ill, recovering from surgery and illness, is usually not in a place of power. Having a caring, trusted advocate who is with the patient can be a powerful agent of healing and recovery.

The role of probiotics within a hospital can be very important. But expect that your physician may not know about the importance, nor believe in it. Talk about probiotics before your surgery if possible. Be aware that it can take 18 years or more before "new discoveries" become integrated into mainstream medicine.

Hospital choices: Recently a relative had a hip replacement. Within her city's hospital systems, the major hospital had a smaller and separate facility just for scheduled orthopedic operations. While the main hospital also did replacements, the smaller, specialized facility had a much lower complication rate, lower infection rate and overall better outcomes. It can take work to find the best option. One simple question a patient can ask doctors and nurses: "If it was your parent/spouse/child, where would you recommend they have surgery?" Then listen for a heartfelt response.

An integrated **team** approach to surgical care that includes increased movement is better for the patient, decreases pain and improves functional outcomes. The University of Pennsylvania School of Medicine recently published an "Enhanced Recovery after Surgery" (ERAS) protocol to reduce the amount of opiate pain medications used after spinal surgery. Their ERAS protocol involves coordination among the entire clinical team—including the surgeons, anesthesiologists, nurses and outpatient staff—so patients can recover safely and with attention to all aspects of their care, not just the surgery. Among other things the protocol called for patients to be up and moving regularly 3–5 times a day, starting the day after surgery. This improved blood flow encouraged healing and decreased the use of narcotic pain medications.

Definition of Recovery Room: After a surgery, the patient is moved to the "Recovery Room" for a brief period, and then moved to a hospital room, or perhaps discharged from the hospital. **Leaving the "Recovery Room" does not mean that the patient has recovered. It means that they are stable enough to be transferred.** The effects of anesthesia can persist for days, weeks and months. Leaving the Recovery Room doesn't mean the patient is "back to normal."

All This Beauty Just for Me

I stand at the edge of the ocean, feel my
mother earth's beating heart.
I am one with my creation, one with the
Creator, and know my special part.
All this beauty just for me; waves of
beauty, as far as eye can see.
I know it's there for all creation equally,
but in this moment, right now
All this beauty is just for me.

"I stand at the edge of abundance,
tune in to the flowing force.
I plunge into the flow, let God, let go;
have faith in my loving Source.
All this bounty just for me; I am master of everything I see.
I know that health and wealth are there to make
me free, and in this moment, right now,
All this bounty is just for me.

When I open my eyes I find beauty, when
I step out in faith I find joy.
When I trust my Source I have bountiful
supply, and a wonder no fear can destroy.

I can stand at the edge of contentment,
turn loose of my fear-filled ways.
I let go of the sadness, know true gladness,
find joy has lightened my days.
All this blessing just for me, I am now serenity.
I find my truth and know the truth can make
me free, and in this moment, right now,
All this blessing is just for me."

Words and music by Noah Karrasch

9

Rebuilding and Rehabilitating Self after Surgery

DAN'S STORY

So, I trusted my physician greatly, and trust in one's physician contributes to the healing process! Recovery from surgery wasn't easy, or quick, or fun, but it was accomplished. Recovery wasn't really painful, but it lasted longer due to the Range of Motion (ROM) restrictions of the posterior approach which I had chosen, based in my trust on the physician I used. I persisted, and happily I'm far along the road to complete recovery.

As a physical therapist, I was faithful to the movement therapies prescribed to me, but also to the wise use of my own body that came from my training. For the most part, both the outside prescriptions and my own thoughts were based on common sense: I didn't overdo, or move too fast, or overwork any of the movements. I faithfully charted all the meds and supplements I was meant to take, as at first the pain was so intense that I was never sure whether I was on schedule unless I wrote things down to ease my mind.

I did allow myself to move into and through the pain, but **I also allowed myself to explore and appreciate the pain, as something that was leading me to my own healing.** This is difficult to explain, but **it seemed, and seems, to me, that it's important to allow one's**

pain to be the guiding influence. I'd advise you, after a surgery, to listen to, respect and humor your body when it suggests it's time to get up, time to stay down and time to eat, drink, relax, move, sleep and heal. Take charge of your own process: Listen to all the advice you want, but listen even more closely to your inner guidance, and you'll find your way back to health.

That Was a Tremendous Insult to Your Body!

So now surgery is past. Perhaps you're still lying in a hospital bed, feeling poorly. The first and biggest advice is simply, still, *relax*. Yes, you're in pain, and it may feel unendurable. You can do this, you will do this. Allow yourself to know you're going to survive. As Dan says, let your pain be the guiding influence. It's not a bad thing to feel pity for self when in pain; but it's more productive to acknowledge the pain and try to keep moving forward through it. Don't beat yourself up if you can't overcome pain. Do give yourself strokes when you can make even small movements or forget your pain even for a few seconds. And remember, hopefully you haven't set your expectations of recovery so high as to set yourself up to fail when you don't heal "fast enough"! You heal when you heal.

After Dr. One's pre-surgery visit with me, during which he made it sound quite routine and as easy as or easier than the first surgery, I thought I was prepared to come in and take the whole drama at a run. Wrong! I was laid so low, I wasn't sure I ever wanted to get out of bed again. One day, at about day three or four in the hospital, it took 20 minutes to talk myself into trying to even sit up and get out of bed. I made it to the edge of the bed, in sitting posture; then decided I really didn't need to see vertical that day, after all. It's got to be OK if you can't do everything you think you should do, or want to do, right away. It seems to me this is one of the major problems most of us face: that desire to be better, right away. It doesn't always happen!

It's so easy to focus on the hurt, the pain, the fear. It's more difficult, but more productive, to focus on the small victories—sneezing without hurting tremendously—keeping down half a cup of tea walking to the door of the room on your own—getting out of bed, or even into a sitting position, unassisted.

This last surgery took me far down, to the point where I wasn't sure I wanted to push back and try to get on my feet again. I truly wasn't sure I wanted to stay alive. It happens! I understand how one can give up—when things hurt so much, it's all you can do to lay around and groan and wish some magic pill would make things all right. For what seemed like a long time, I hurt too much to really try. The road can seem too long and too rough, and you can feel it would be easier to surrender and allow others to bring you along, or to just let go and stop trying. If you expect others to carry you across the finish line, you'll have a much harder recovery. But if you can convince yourself that tiny steps are the way to get started, you'll finish much faster.

You must be in charge of the process: You can develop the team, but healing will happen much faster if you see yourself as the captain of that team. The doctor may be the quarterback, but you are the captain and the coach, if you'll accept the job.

> It's so easy to focus on the hurt, the pain, the fear. It's more difficult, but more productive, to focus on the small victories.

So even at this stage, asking questions, seeking explanations and getting answers you need are appropriate behaviors. Though medical personnel are paid to get you better, they're not paid to care. Some, many, do care, but, truly, no one can care for you like you can care for yourself.

Realize that I write about my personal experience, and you may not have an experience anything like mine. Most of my ideas will serve you...especially if you adapt them to your situation. For example, if you're having a hip or knee replacement, you're basically a well person at this time, and, though recovery may be long and involved, with pain, it's a different situation. An operation to trim a disc or remove a lamina in the spine is far different from what I've experienced. A surgery to open your heart cavity and make changes inside isn't similar to my spinal or stomach surgeries. But the same rules apply: Take care of yourself, get the information you can get before you go under the knife, stay relaxed, and remember both to move but also to take care of yourself after the fact.

Be in Charge: Grounded Connection

Don't be afraid to ask for help! And don't be afraid to be loud if help doesn't come. Years ago, after the extensive orthopedic and neurosurgery to repair plane wreck damage, due to all the pain meds I'd been offered and accepted, I hadn't had a bowel movement for a month. Imagine that! One day the doctor decided it was time to get rid of the urinary catheter as well, so told me to drink lots of fluids so I'd "make water." Well, after hours of drinking fluids and having no bowel activity for a month, I was miserable. When asking for help, I was told the doctor's orders were to keep the catheter out until I urinated on my own power. Finally, I couldn't stand the pain anymore, and began yelling…at the top of my lungs! I just screamed in pain, as loudly as I could.

Guess what? Several attendants showed up immediately, made a call to the doctor, got a catheter reinstalled (and found my bladder was so full as to be dangerous), and eventually even provided an enema which helped but didn't totally relieve the pressure. I'd heard in the past that cranky patients usually get better because they don't mind expressing their needs, but this was the first time I explored that territory. I'm less shy about expressing myself these days.

After this same early surgery, on the second night after the operation a temporary nurse who'd not seen me before came to check my vital signs at 2 am. She found my temperature was a bit high, probably 100.4 or some such number—certainly not a horrible number for 36 hours post-surgery. She immediately called my doctor for instructions as to what should be done. The doc wasn't on duty, so his "partner," who was covering and knew nothing about me or my case, told her, "I don't think it's anything to worry about, but just to be sure (what I call CYA medicine, see below) let's give him an upright chest X-ray to see he's clear of pneumonia." An upright chest X-ray? I'm in a hospital bed, with a broken spine, a long surgery scar with two-day-old seven-inch long Harrington rods anchored in my spine, not supposed to move at all, haven't been vertical in over a week, and you want me to have an *upright* X-ray?

After discerning the futility of trying to get me upright, the attendants painfully rolled me around in my bed, put some kind of film plate under me, took their X-ray, and came back within an hour. They told me the plate was out of focus and inconclusive so they were going through the procedure again. At this point my common sense kicked in; I said, "No, you're not going to do that." They needed that simple turndown from me that allowed them to have fulfilled their instructions…they had CYA'd—Covered Their A _ _es—and could chart that I'd taken responsibility away from them. What a learning: I realized I could refuse any procedure or drug, and the professionals could then chart that I'd assumed responsibility and taken it from their shoulders. I see this as reclaiming control, and to me it was important.

This is an ongoing and critical piece that we all need to understand. CYA medicine is rampant! So many doctors are wary of lawsuits for malpractice…if they don't prescribe every test they can think of that may or may not have anything to do with a person's condition, they might miss the test that will catch a problem. It's far easier to order that every possibility be tested, even when common sense suggests all aren't needed. As the patient, you have the right to deny any and all tests if they make no sense to you. For that matter you have the right to deny treatments as well, if treatment feels wrong to you or you don't see its value, or even if you're choosing to give up and quit struggling. Remember, the cranky patient gets better!

> I realized I could refuse any procedure or drug, and the professionals could then chart that I'd assumed responsibility and taken it from their shoulders.

Know what someone wants to do to you, why, what results they're expecting, and how this process helps your overall healing. If you don't get the answers you want, keep digging, or find someone who can give you answers.

It's common sense that CYA medicine contributes greatly to the skyrocketing cost of medical care. If a doctor feels the need to prescribe every test imaginable to make sure he's ruled out every possible diagnosis, think how many of those procedures are expensive and potentially could be avoided! Think carefully when your doctor wants ever more tests, and feel all right about saying "no."

An interesting aside: Studies show that doctors with good communication skills are sued for malpractice far less frequently than doctors who don't know how to or won't talk with their patients. Even when outcomes are bad, those patients and families who feel they've been made part of the team and are advised *and* consulted, don't tend to sue. When patients and families feel heard, they tend to be more forgiving. Likewise, research now shows that though doctors used to be afraid to apologize or accept blame for "mistakes," these days doctors who fearlessly face patients and families to admit mistakes are forgiven most of the time.[1] Patients—and their families—simply want to be heard, acknowledged, cared about and treated as a person, not a condition.

---

1   Gatti, Keltner, Bienvenu & Montesi (2013) "Research: Doctors, Patients Benefit When Doctors Apologize." Accessed on 22/5/2019 at www.gkbm.com/blog/2013/february/research-doctors-patients-benefit-when-doctors-a.

In this last hospital visit, I began the "incarceration" in a double room with a very nice man in the far bed. We both had IV machines which beep warnings for various problems: a clog in the IV, running out of a fluid, a nose plug that registers insufficient air intake or a dying battery are a few examples of what might get such a machine beeping. On our second night together, about every ten minutes one of our machines began the loud, steady beeping that woke both of us. We'd call a nurse to reset a machine. Usually somewhere within the next 15 minutes someone would come, push one button and we'd be on our own again…only to get back to sleep and have the machine begin its warnings again, nearly immediately! Neither of us could get rest.

Since my machine seemed to complain more of the time, I finally told my nurse I'd prefer to live without the IV pain meds so as to not have to listen to it! I had her disconnect me from the "on demand" pain meds so I could get sleep. Waking every ten minutes was more painful than feeling the regular pain. On the last day of my stay, one nurse finally told me that often the IV monitoring machine needed a simple reset and showed me how to push one button. After seven days of being awakened by and upset with that silly machine, I learned that I could reset it myself. Why didn't I think to ask for that bit of power much sooner?

And on that final day of the seven long days and nights, a new nurse gave me a regularly scheduled anticoagulant shot in the stomach. Whether it was the sitting position I was in, her style or something I can't identify…I only know hers was the most brutal shot I'd *ever* experienced…every other such shot over the seven days was a mild tiny prick; this one felt like I'd been stabbed. I immediately yelled out loud; then told her that she'd just given the absolute worst shot of the entire stay. Later that day, she came to give another round of the same shot. I asked if I could refuse and she told me, yes, of course. Immediately I refused, and I survived and thrived by taking back that small bit of my power.

Power is an interesting concept here. In a hospital bed, recovering, in pain, mentally confused by both pain and the drugs that mask it, you're reasonably powerless. A doctor, nurse or assistant can come and tell you what's going to happen, and you may or may not have the faculties to consider whether what they're saying is valid. This is another reason it's always good to have that "advocate"—a family member or friend who can sit with you, help you think through the questions you may have for your doctor or caregiver, help you find the call button when it's gone missing or a sip of water when the cup is just out of reach, and in general make sure you're as comfortable as possible so you can focus on healing. When no one else is there to advocate for you, it's difficult, but possible, to take charge of your own process. In my surgeries, I've had some successes and some failures. I'm choosing, now, to see those failures as learning experiences for me. Hospital staff members aren't required to like you; they are hired to serve you. You're certainly paying for the privilege of being there, and your health is their product. Expect them to deliver a good product to you.

Time to Feel Better! Self-Regulation

Let's talk about ways you can push yourself gently to accomplish more even while hurting. If I realize, and believe, that pain is resistance to change, then I begin to realize how, when it hurts to move, I choose to quit moving. But, as Dan says, we can allow pain to be the guiding influence.

In the "old days" one stayed in the hospital bed for up to a week before getting up and moving. We now realize that moving more quickly enhances healing…and often, in fact, one is gotten out of bed within hours of a surgery. Yes, it will hurt— you will hurt. But if you can breathe, relax and explore the pain calmly instead of bracing against it, you heal faster. Let's begin thinking about ways to move, breathe, explore so that you can acknowledge, then conquer the pain and fear associated with surgery. Consider these ideas:

- Realize you've been assaulted! Consider that you've been bruised, not only inside, but outside as well, and be OK with taking time to heal. One of our biggest problems is our impatience. Remember, you took a deep insult; take time to allow that insult to be healed. Too often we have the feeling that things need to be better right away. **Don't feel you must bounce back quickly or do too much too fast.** Pain can be seen as fear of or resistance to feeling— both your body's pains, but also emotional pain…and these two are quite wrapped in each other. Can you challenge yourself to feel the pain, in appropriate doses, and allow it to deliver its message and move on through you?

- Find a reason to get better. I literally had many reasons this last time but was hurting so much I couldn't stay focused on them. Accept that you may have some dark days but think of some reward down the path that makes you want to at least try a bit.

- Visitors: Proceed with caution! Depending on how severe your surgery has been, how close a relationship you have with someone, how contagious you are and how much alone time you crave, you may choose to limit visitors. Generally, on this past hospital stay of one week, I didn't want or encourage visitors, and let my friends know that prayers from afar were more helpful than visits from outside. On the day of surgery one friend sat in the waiting room, then came and sat in my hospital room for a few hours, saying nothing but only being a supportive presence. She was very welcome and very healing for me. Shortly after, I realized that gathering the energy to say hello and carrying on conversation was just too much work for me. I put out the word that I'd prefer to heal alone. Then, I found that, with C. *diff* and being highly contagious, I didn't want friends being exposed as well. Choose if and whether you're ready for visitors and be all right with limiting those visits. True friends and caring family will understand your wishes, and there's absolutely nothing wrong with alone time if it heals you.

My roommate for several days had many visitors. It was clear from listening in to conversations that he was a good and caring man. His wife was there much of the time, probably 6–8 hours a day, and I didn't mind hearing their conversations. But on the day I was sickest, he received a visit from a woman I'd describe as an emotional vampire...she seemed to suck all the energy and strength from the room. Signs posted in the hospital advised visitors to stay 20 minutes or less; she stayed five hours! In that time, she never stopped talking, in a whiny, sing-song voice, about all her problems. I found myself listening, hearing his non-committal, semi-counseling responses to her chatter, and found myself getting angry, wanting to ask her to be quiet. I didn't interfere with that horrible visit, other than to get earplugs, until hour four; but I truly feel her energy made me far less well. Today, I would confront the problem and set healthy boundaries much earlier. I've learned that lesson.

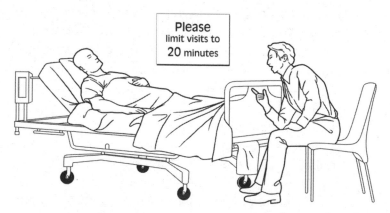

Don't feel the need to "entertain" visitors; take care of yourself!

- Remember, if possible, to find an "advocate" to run interference for you when you're overwhelmed. This concept is even more important once you've come through the surgery. Whether you need someone to be your cheerleader when you're feeling blue, or someone to nudge you when you allow yourself to feel too negative, or someone to listen to the professional staff and ask and get answers to hard questions and answers, or even someone to do all of these things when the time is appropriate, the more you find that trusted ear, and use it, the better you'll be able to move the unprocessed thoughts and feelings, which contributes to moving energy in all ways, and enhancing healing.

- Pay attention to what you eat! Revisit the chart of poisons, and realize how many of the poisonous foods, especially sugar, are pervasive in much of what's served in hospital.

- Remember also: You are your final authority. See your doctors, nurses, family as the team…listen to all the advice but listen to your gut as well. Perhaps this surgery is an opportunity to accept help and positive energy from others? Explore this concept too. I realized, strongly, during my surgery 30 years ago that I'd been a giver for too long, and the trauma let me learn to accept healing from others instead of giving it all the time. It was hard to be brought so low, but it was a great lesson and learning for me.

Too often doctors have a certain model and mindset. Without making them wrong, add a bit of your own rehab skills to their treatment plan. What's YOUR treatment plan? Make decisions about your doctor's recommendations but see their ideas as just that—recommendations.

To Medicate, or Not to Medicate? Fuel, or Poison?

For example, do you really need two pain medications? Sleeping pills? All these can be good, but also hard on the liver and can slow down the digestive system, which is the last fellow to return to you anyway. Honor your digestive system by trying to stay away from overmedication. It's quite easy to push that little button that puts more pain medication into your system. However, that very medication dramatically slows down both digestive and eliminative functions as a by-product. How do you balance the need for pain medications with the fact that they also slow down the healing process? This is a difficult balance to keep. I've been told since this last surgery that doctors are now beginning to move away from these "on demand" medications, and I think that's a healthy step. It's easy to abuse pain meds when you're in pain! Sadly, much of our country can attest to the truth of this statement; witness the opioid epidemic in our country today.

And keep in mind that some of the prescribed medication can still be seen as CYA meds…if a doctor doesn't try every option and explore, just as with tests, s/he is more liable to receive a lawsuit suggesting they've not done all they should do. You may well be prescribed pain meds, stool softeners, anticoagulants and more, whether you need them or not. Do you feel you need them? Are you willing to talk to your doctor about your concerns?

At age 78 my mother had a nasty bout with the shingles virus, which lasted quite a long while. She went to hospital with the pain and was immediately given a drug that was meant to soothe it. It made her sick to her stomach, so she was given another med for stomach pain that made her crazy. At this stage, her doctor told us, her guardians, that it was necessary to remove her gall bladder!

I'd been reading up in the PDF or *Physician's Desk Reference,* which lists uses, properties and side effects of any drug on the market…the first medication given had a side effect of stomach upset, and the second had an effect of mental confusion. I was fairly sure this underweight older woman was being overmedicated. I confronted her doctor directly: "Are you telling me her meds aren't contributing to the problem?" He assured me that they couldn't be the problem, even though I knew they were! I responded: "Here's what we're going to do... no surgery. I want her weaned from those meds in the reverse order of how they were put in; then let's see who she is and how she feels." On letting go of the drugs, her mind cleared, then her stomach was no longer upset, and she only had the shingles pain. This seemed a far better solution than losing a gall bladder, which wouldn't have made any difference, I believe. In fact, that trauma could easily have killed her.

And, interestingly, at the time my 78-year-old mother said to us: "Don't talk to that doctor about what you're thinking; he might get mad at me and make things worse." She was in such tremendous pain and mental confusion that she couldn't make good choices; we were lucky to be there for her. After the situation was resolved, she admitted we probably saved her life by questioning the doctor's intentions. She lived another ten reasonably happy years before being injured in an accident that eventually contributed to her demise.

I'm not opposed to taking medications; I'm just opposed to blindly taking them because they're in front of you. Most of us need pain meds, especially, in the first days. But remembering these pills are a crutch; do you want to live on crutches forever? Or are you ready to try to step out on your own, sooner?

Often, I tell a new client that if her fibromyalgia pain is intense and she can't get good sleep, I think sleeping pills make sense. Clients are relieved to hear this from someone in the "alternative" community. But it's true; **I'm not opposed to medications; I'm opposed to overmedication.** While I understand the damage done to the liver by medications, sometimes something as simple as restful sleep seems more important. In fact, some hospitals are beginning to experiment with less night-time interventions on patients (vital sign measurements, etc.) so as to give patients better sleep, and are seeing positive results from more restful nights. Common sense prevails, sometimes!

Will You Be Scarred for Life?

Scars will necessarily be the result of your surgery…there's no way you can receive cuts and not be scarred. However, there are ideas to consider both before the surgery, but especially after. Scars may stay for life, but they don't have to control your life forever.

First, let's consider what may be called a "keyhole" surgery. Realize that, even though the outer scar may be tiny, the deeper inside the surgeon has traveled, the more tissues have been interrupted. What may seem a tiny scar may be hiding a tremendous amount of trauma! The size of the scar doesn't necessarily tell you how invasive and damaging that surgery has been. And you may have no sense of which muscles, which meridians and, sadly, which nerves have been cut in the surgical process.

My last surgery, which repaired the colostomy surgery which was required nearly 30 years after my plane wreck, was difficult: The first surgery's scar of 6 inches was cut out and expanded to 10 inches, from pubic bone to just below the sternum. Think of the layers involved! In addition to skin and superficial fascia, many sets of muscles were cut before reaching into the abdominal cavity to "rip" the colon away from the spleen so as to shorten and reattach it to the rectum. I felt horribly abused, and still feel a degree of the abuse to this day. Recently I've had scar work from one of my students, and can attest to the idea that good, slow, intentional work to release the layers of scarring and adhesions caused by the scalpel can restore function to tissue that simply feels either dead or damaged. If you've had severe surgery, working with a bodyworker who's trained in scar tissue release work can be literally freeing.

Years ago, at one of the first dissection courses I attended, I asked the professor, "What causes adhesions?" Adhesions are the internal shortening and tightening of tissues that seem to have decided to glue themselves together in response to some stress. Her response: We think it's caused by the tissues being exposed to air." While this is a valid explanation, why do some people have adhesions who've never had surgery? My common-sense answer is that some of us tend to live our lives in a shortened, fearful, move-forward-carefully posture and attitude. If that's the case, clearly the more we can move and stretch internally, either on our own or with the assistance of someone trained to release such holding patterns, the healthier we'll be.

So, whether you have scarring and adhesions from your surgery, or whether you just feel like a tense and tight person overall, deep tissue bodywork from a therapist trained to work with such stuck tissues makes sense.

And We're Back to Breath and Movement

Let's revisit breath work. So many people don't bother to find the places that hurt and then try to accept breath, calmly going into that pain, to try to go through it. Once out of the hospital, I thought perhaps I had a mild case of pneumonia, as I couldn't seem to get a deep breath. My brother-in-law, Dr. Harvey, suggested I might be experiencing allergies, so prescribed an allergy med and a bronchial dilator inhaler. On the very first inhale from that dilator, I could feel the lungs opening, but what I felt even more strongly was that I hadn't been breathing deeply because it hurt too much! Once I owned this, I was able to focus on getting deeper breaths and starting to move energy down to the pain.

Years ago a friend fell off her roof and broke her back. I was the first call she made, and immediately went to her ER bedside. She asked me to take her into a meditation to deal with the pain. I took her *into* her pain, not away from it. Short term, she felt further damaged, but long term, she healed very well. I'd had a similar situation back during my plane wreck. When the medical team finally realized I wasn't giving permission for surgery immediately, they left me alone. Finally, by myself, I realized I could no longer find a deep breath. I spent 30–60 minutes just working to put breath down into my painful back. I wonder: If I hadn't chosen to work for that breath, would I be walking today? Or would I still be paralyzed?

Nausea: It happens. The more you can take deep breaths (in itself a tremendous challenge at this time) the less it will bother you. Vomiting may happen as well, particularly if you've had a tube down your throat as part of the anesthesia process; this tube may have damaged your throat and made you susceptible to vomiting. Warning: Avoid powdered broths such as vegetable or beef. On day two that powdered creation went down badly and came up horribly painfully!

After a surgery you'll obviously spend lots of time simply lying in the hospital bed. Scoot down in the bed so your feet can touch its footboard. Push gently with one foot, with breath; then the other, with breath. Explore and stay awhile. Can you find that simple pressure in the foot translating up your body into the place where you've been violated surgically? Can you allow yourself to explore that connection between the feet and legs and the trauma? Can you find, explore, and add breath and movement? Simply lie on the bed and slowly drag one heel, allowing your knee to rise toward the ceiling. If possible, keep your low back down as well. Foot and leg exercises in bed, done gently, aren't really that hard!

Consider shutting off the news, for sure, and possibly the entire television as well, other than your favorite shows or the "relaxation channel" if your hospital offers one. Limit TV time. Explore reading, working easy puzzles, feeling your body, listening to music. Know your attention span may not be great but give yourself credit; you're coming back from an assault! Essence of time is your best medicine. It's OK to be pretty lazy.

Stretching is useful; just don't overdo it. Allow yourself to again look for the places that don't want to be felt and invite them to soften. Even in bed, one can move the legs, twist the body side to side, turn to one side or another, roll the head and neck around, shrug the shoulders. We all know how after a surgery it hurts to move; we know too that if we don't move, there will be far more scar tissue, shortening of connective tissues and muscles, and more problems in the long run. Move slowly, but move.

Pay attention to your posture! It's so easy to lie in bed with lots of pillows propping you up, but pillows also shorten the front of your body's sitting posture, for example, adding to the surgery trauma. After a stomach or heart surgery we often try to keep that insulted area shortened, so as to not stretch or challenge the painful tissue. Remember to visit the insult, slowly and carefully. Try to shift postures; explore keeping your neck long and head on straight, and periodically check in to stay aware. A knee or hip surgery will often suggest to you "Just don't move that part." Move it, but slowly, carefully, with intention. Be aware! Frozen shoulders or frozen anything comes often because someone hears their doctor tell them to not move that joint. A bit of exploration is always good; too much is usually not good. Pain can be your guiding influence, but not your boss!

> Stretching is useful; just don't overdo it. Allow yourself to again look at the places that say they don't want to be felt and invite them to soften. Even in bed, one can move the legs, twist the body side to side, turn to one side or another, roll the head and neck around, shrug the shoulders.

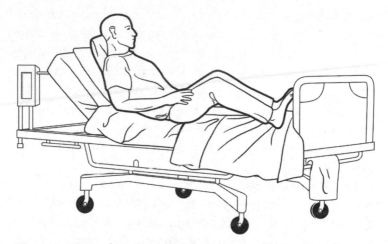

Pay attention to the way you're allowing yourself to sit, lie and stand.

My wife recently had an elbow replacement; an old fall had given her a silicone spacer for 40 years, and it had worn out over time. Her physical therapist in her only visit told her she was at the top of the heap in terms of healing and movement, but warned her not to go too fast or too furiously. He told her of another super patient who had lifted too much, too early, and ripped out the entire process so she had to have the same surgery a second time. We can try to do too much, too early, if we're not aware.

When you're able to sit in a chair, place your arms/elbows on the chair arms and just explore lifting yourself out of the chair. You don't even have to lift; just explore reclaiming a bit of arm and shoulder strength. Sitting and lying around takes your muscle tone away quickly. How can you regain a bit of tone? Remember Chapter 5, which encouraged you to use any and every piece of furniture and physical features of your room or house as exercise equipment? Let getting in and out of bed become an exercise; let lifting up and down from a chair be part of your workout routine; let walking slowly and with intention to the bathroom be exercise. When you're ready to sit, remember to work to sit in front of your sitting bones instead of behind them, thus straightening the entire spine and allowing freedom and movement up and down it. And remember to breathe into and acknowledge your pain.

Slow walking is fine! These days, often you're out of bed on the day of many surgeries, or nearly always by the next day. The first walk may be only as far as sitting up, or standing and taking a step or two, but it's important to begin moving. Without shoes, gripper stockings are best (hospitals usually provide them). Really work to slow down the walk, explore and feel every part of each foot touch the floor, and see how your body responds when various "hiding" places start to appear. When I first stepped back into my left foot, I could feel it wanting to "protect" my splenic area where there'd been such an insult to the tissue as they freed the colon from the spleen. Knowing I was trying to protect that line, I focused on putting a bit of weight into and through it; I could feel myself return to that part of my body.

When you're ready to walk, IVs, catheters and other equipment can get in your way. Work around them, gratefully and without needing to cut or throw them away. You'll be excited on the day you can walk without your beanpole IV friend. Perhaps a friend can come for your daily walk or walks, and drag along your equipment for you, until you're able to move it yourself.

Common sense is usually the best course. Allow yourself to use it. You know your doctor may be in charge in this setting, but you're driving the vehicle that he or she is restoring, and you know your vehicle better than anyone outside it. Listen to it, observe it, take care of it. Give it appropriate physical and mental fuels. Maintain it, oil it with movement and water. Simply choosing to see this insult to your body as a necessary setback, from which you can and will come back, can give you the strength to move forward instead of giving up.

There's No Place Like Home!

Nearly all of us feel better, simply by getting out of hospital. Once you're released, you're on your own, and it can be a blessing and a curse. Perhaps you'll need someone around to fetch and serve; perhaps you'll be able to take care of yourself. For me this is always a major goal; I don't like being dependent on the kindness of others...I want to take care of myself. And perhaps this is one of my big lessons. It was clear to me back in 1987 when I had the plane wreck and a month of hospitalization that one of my lessons was just that: to learn to receive from others instead of giving endlessly to others. So, accept help, and even learn to ask for it. What's your lesson, beyond the physical repair? Do you need to learn to accept help and love? Do you simply need to learn to take care of the body you've been given? Ask for the message, listen and wait...it will come.

We have a small and loving circle of friends who want to be helpful. The day I was leaving the hospital from this last surgery, I emailed them all, asking for help! This was a new and novel idea for me. My wonderful friends all responded quickly and positively, and it was a blessing both to me that they were there, but also to them that they could feel helpful and supportive as true friends want to be. Ask for what you need and keep asking until you find the help you want. In addition to my "asks," often they volunteered their love and service in ways I hadn't considered. What a blessing to have such a network! And think about it: Most friends want to be helpful, so why shouldn't you ask for what you need from them that allows them to be the helpful friend they want to be for you? Wouldn't you want to do the same for them?

Is your bed high enough, or too high? Can you make it to the toilet on your own? Can you prepare foods for yourself, or do you need someone to be with you all the time? Most of us just want to get on with it and do for ourselves, but it's OK to need help from others, and to accept it.

At home one can also really focus on healing. What else do you have to do but get better? Allow yourself to take a few more days off work and focus on your stamina returning. Again, the slow and steady pace of healing will get you back to your routine much quicker than overdoing whatever you think must happen right away. Essence of time remains one of your better medicines.

It really is easy to get lazy when dealing with the sort of trauma you've been through over the course of treatment. Once you feel a bit better, it's a simple matter to "skip" a day or two of the walking, the healthy eating, the exercise routine. It's easy to think, "Just one small piece of wedding cake…" or "I deserve a day off from all that thinking about getting better." Be aware: You can never stop expending the energy required to stay healthy. Once you begin sliding down that slope, it's more and more difficult to pick back up and move forward again. Choose to take small steps if necessary; but keep moving forward.

Once at home, it's an interesting balance you seek, between pushing yourself to heal and remembering to give yourself time to regain strength by resting. You'll find your balance by remembering to honor your bodymindcore as you come back to your normal life. Take the time you need, even if you don't think you have it…if you don't let yourself recover slowly but steadily, you may set yourself back and need to start from square one again, and that's not pleasant. Realize that once you begin to feel better, unless you pace yourself you'll be tempted to let go of the new and helpful patterns and get back to what you've done in the past. Don't. Allow yourself to remain in a slower, more meditative state where you're paying attention to what you do and who you've become.

LAST WORDS FROM THE DOCTOR

In general, I think for every one day someone is in hospital, it can take at least one week to recover. Often patients expect that they will be "back to normal" within a few days of a surgery.

We can talk about the person having at least five sides: Physical, Emotional, Intellectual, Spiritual, and the Integrative Mind. All five parts are "injured" in hospital, and all five require time and space to recover.

Pain is a major issue for most patients after surgery. For decades, the US health care model relied on narcotic pain medications after surgery. In 2017 a movement began to reduce the number of narcotics given to patients for pain. However, the focus for most doctors is still: Give a prescription, give a pill. Many patients will have a hard time getting free from narcotics. **Studies released in 2018 and 2019 show that for Emergency Room (ER) patients, tylenol/acetaminophen or non-steroidal drugs like motrin/ibuprofen or aleve/naprosyn can be just as effective as a narcotic.**[2] The potential for addiction to and dependence on narcotics cannot be understated.

For most patients, their experience after surgery is passive: lying in bed, attended by nurses and doctors who keep asking about and focusing on patient pain. Too often overlooked or ignored are some of the "other" foundations to healing which include movement, breathing and mindfulness. Old truism: We will get what we focus on. If our focus is pain, then medication is an easy and quick relief. If we focus on movement, breathing and mindfulness, then pain is only one of the areas of our surgical/hospital experience

Noah's description of visitors who drain the patient's energy is, if anything, understated. I once had a patient who had just delivered her first child and was very anxious to breastfeed. Her own anxiety was interfering with her ability to "let down" and let the milk flow. Making

---

2   E.E. Krebs *et al.* (2018) "Effect of opioid vs nonopioid medications on pain-related function in patients with chronic back pain or hip or knee osteoarthritis pain: The SPACE randomized clinical trial." *JAMA 319*, 9, 872–882.

it worse was the constant surrounding by at least six friends and relatives all "cheering her on" to breastfeed. The more they tried to act as a cheering squad, the more tense the patient became. By the time I acted as her advocate, and had the nurse kick all the relatives out, the damage was already done. Being surrounded by a group of people who have their own expectations and "demands" for the patient rarely brings health or encouragement.

Keep in mind the importance of the autonomic nervous system and our need for balance between the sympathetic (fight, flee or freeze) and parasympathetic (relax) systems. Sympathetic is alert, aroused, on guard and ready for fight, flee or freeze responses. Parasympathetic is rest, recovery and recharge. This concept of balance is often ignored or overlooked in our traditional Western model of medicine. Hospital and surgical decisions are often designed to encourage the sympathetic side and often ignore the parasympathetic side. Too often, patients are forced to make decisions while caught up in an overwhelmed wave of alert/on guard/ crisis messages and thinking. They decide on surgery in a framework of sympathetic overload: overwhelmed, afraid and alone. The natural response is to trust that authority figure, usually the doctor. The relationship becomes unbalanced as the patient is surrounded by fear. Sympathetic alert is great for a brief "emergency or crisis," but it's the relaxation, rest and remaining in a place of trust and safety (again, the parasympathetic side) that allows the body to recover and heal. Being always on edge, always on alert, interferes with healing.

Final Thoughts

As I've admitted throughout this book, I teach what I need to learn, and I've honestly tried to show you in these pages how I've made quite a few mistakes on my own journey over the years. I continue to see those mistakes as learning experiences; both for me and for the clients who cross my path in the future. So, maybe there really are no mistakes. Maybe I had to take wrong turns so I could better direct others to a clearer path.

And that path is so full of common sense. Most of us truly know many things we could be doing to make our lives and bodymindcores happier and better functioning…and most of us choose to ignore those very things. It really is this simple (note, *not* this easy!): We could move more often, fill our systems with healthy physical, mental and emotional fuels, take charge of our own processes instead of handing our power to others, find reasons to feel joyful and on purpose and search for a balanced state in our life. If we followed these guidelines, chances are we'd manage to prevent many of the surgeries we feel are necessary, and even live longer, happier and more fulfilled lives. Remember, whether you think you can or you can't, you're right. Do you think you can change your world for the better?

> You can never stop expending the energy required to stay healthy. Once you begin sliding down that slope, it's more and more difficult to pick back up and move forward again. Choose to take small steps if necessary; but keep moving forward.

I invite you to explore health, to explore better self-care: freer motion, more nutritious fuels, feelings of safety in your world, calm in your own nervous system and happier thoughts in healthier relationships. Balancing the five principles of self-regulation (head), social connection (heart), nutrition (gut), relaxation (groin) and movement (extremities) can allow you to choose health over sickness, joy over sadness or anger, purpose over overwhelm and common sense over someone else's prescription for you. You can do it! Many others have, and you will too. The question is, will you explore health, or choose to be overwhelmed by sickness? Remember, you don't have to do everything overnight, and you may or may not ever get back to the fullness of the life you had, but you can be grateful for the life you have. Get to work, get back on your feet, be gentle with yourself, but don't let yourself give up! Good luck!

Whether you picked up this book because you were facing a surgery, dealing with the after-effects, or wanting to keep surgery at bay…in any of these situations, movement, breath and positive attitude of gratitude will go a long way in helping you feel better. I wish, for you, health, freedom and joy.

Be blessed, live fully, and may you continue to evolve into a healthy and happy soul on this planet.

Quick Reference Guide to Mindful Movements

One of the most important and simple (not easy!) postural cues and awareness ideas we could benefit from planting into our bodymindcore comes from Dr. Ida Rolf, creator of Rolfing or Structural Integration. She used to suggest to clients and students that they simply learn to stay in a totally upright posture by keeping head up and waist back at the same time.

I've refined this idea in my own practice, by suggesting that clients and students be aware of the four major centers of the body: head, heart, gut and groin, and do all they can to keep the four centers both further apart, but also in straighter alignment. Thus, keeping head upback makes sense, as does keeping waist back. But why not focus on leading with the heart as well? Why not ask the groin to pull downforward, while the waist pulls upback, while the heart leads, while the head stay on top? See *An All Purpose Cue* for this head up/waist back idea revisited. Below we'll look at specific centers of the body and a handy reference to tell you where to revisit if you're most interested in bringing energy to the head, or heart, or gut or groin.

Head/Neck
Among the problems we might find in the head and neck: headaches, tumors, temporomandibular joint problems (TMJ), anxiety, panic disorders, insomnia, overall pain through the

body, "fogginess" in the brain, mental illnesses, memory and dementia issues, shoulder problems, as well as sensory problems with vision, smell, hearing, taste, and so on. When the brain is overwhelmed, the body must follow.

I often think of a turtle…when it feels safe, the head pulls out of the shell and the turtle moves through life. As soon as any danger shows itself, that turtle pulls the head, snap! Back into the body. In some ways, I think we've done that to ourselves. I believe if we could simply keep our head up, waist back, and allow the neck to be long and flexible, we'd have far less problems with this head center, because energy could reach it. Explore keeping a long and healthy neck with a "good head on your shoulders." What have you got to lose? In Chapter 6 on movement we focus on a few ways one can open and "oil" this neck to provide better energy to the head. Revisit *Sitting on Those Toes*, *A Good Head on Your Shoulders* and *Still* the *Shoulders*.

Heart Hinge

For years I've suggested to clients that they might experiment with what I call "opening the heart hinge." It seems that between much of the work we do (computing, driving, craft work) and the feeling of emotional protection (early development of height or breasts, childhood emotional abuse or feelings of unworthiness) many of us choose to collapse the area of our chest where our heart lives. Can you see how such a collapse could lead to extra tension in the heart area and put further strain on the muscle? I often suggest someone learn to let their heart be the first center of the body to arrive in any situation. As you think of this idea, can you feel your body reacting by shortening its front face? The exercises *Arms: The Front Legs*, *Hanging from the Front Legs*, *Wrists and Fingers Too* and *Animal Walks* will help you with this idea of keeping an open heart hinge.

In addition to cardiovascular issues, congestive heart failure, atrial fibrillation, aneurisms and other heart issues, this closed heart hinge area can often lead to problems with the lungs and the breath, as well as the head and neck—if the hinge is closed, it suggests we've been collapsing our spine forward. Our control panel and our workhorse have gotten too close together! Whenever energy gets slowed, disease ensues.

Gut

If we go back to the idea that movement helps our body, no matter what our issue, can you see how a bit of movement in the middle of the body could help with digestion and elimination? Between the fact that too many of us eat too much, and too much of really non-nutritive foods, or even "dead" foods, how can we keep health in our gut? In addition to healthy eating, drinking plenty of water instead of our favorite beverages, and considering probiotics and even prebiotics or prebiotic foods, we could also learn to "digest" the emotional traumas that too many of us seem to believe we have to "stomach" as we quietly let them "eat us up" inside.

Any movements will be helpful in keeping the extra weight away from our middle, as will all the above ideas. Particularly helpful: I'd recommend visiting twisting, lateral flexion and forward and back movements as great ways to help keep off the extra pounds and to keep foods moving through you. Return to *Bend, Twist, Flex, Twist and Turn, Side Flexion* and *Now for the Drivers* when you're interested in getting in touch with your "gut" issues.

Groin

I find the body systems most related to this groin element are the reproductive and eliminative systems of the body…those which not only allow our "tight ass" condition to release and resolve, but which also insure the survival of our species.

Conditions which might occur when we have feelings of sexual shaming: overweight, underweight, difficult menstrual cycles, migraine headaches, difficulty in conceiving and delivering, cystitis, fibroid tumors, ovarian or prostrate problems, incontinence or diarrhea, low back and tailbone pain or any other problems which seem to center around the groin area. Can you see how a slowdown of energy, caused by the feelings of shame too many of us have assigned to our sexual nature, could cause such difficulties? Can you allow your sexual energy to flow through your groin, and through you?

It's my theory that most of us are stuck in this groin energy; thus, energy can't rise further, into the gut, heart and head. By simply focusing on bringing breath, energy and awareness into the groin, then asking that energy to rise further into the gut and hopefully higher, we can allow ourselves to be open to an energetic flow throughout the body. I'll often lie on my back, put my hands on my stomach and focus on bringing energy through the groin and towards the gut. On some days I can literally feel the movement beyond the gut, into the heart and occasionally into the head area. I consider this type of breath to be a reset of the vagus mechanism…simply finding energy all the way through the being seems to give the entire bodymindcore a good, deep exhale!

As most of us live in shame in our groin area, these stretches that invite us to open, explore, find/face/feel and forget the shame can make huge changes in our bodymindcore, if we can be open to change. See *Squatting: A Lost Art*, *Opening the Sacroiliac Junctions*, *Underthings: Hamstrings and Adductors*, *Hamstrings Alone* and *An Easier Hamstring Stretch* for ideas that assist the groin in staying open and energized.

Shoulders

Too many of us have troubles with shoulder girdles; we're diagnosed with "rotator cuff injury" and consider the surgery. I believe that sometimes shoulders will repair themselves with simple attention and careful work on our part. Consider especially *Arms: The Front Legs* and *Hanging from the Front Legs* if shoulders are your main problem. Remember the idea brought forth through the entire book: Explore, don't achieve! The concept here is to not further injure or reinjure tissues, but to bring them back to a state of usefulness.

Knees

Likewise, many of us have lost that concept of "use it or lose it" and our knees simply don't want to work anymore. If this is your condition, consider *Squatting: A Lost Art* and working with stairs as your exercise equipment. Use *Big Toe Pushups* and the *Bend and Lift* idea. Remember, in any of these ideas, push yourself gently. It's not necessary to change the world overnight; your body won't change overnight either. Allow yourself to slowly explore movements and you will be rewarded. Push through the pain and you'll be further punished.

Further Resources

I'll divide this reference section into two segments: The first I'll call THINK and the second ACT. In each segment I'll feature books I believe may be helpful if you want to continue your healing process, with a brief description as to why this book may be useful to you. Each list is given in the order of what I consider to be the most helpful book for the section—you may find other books resonate with you more strongly. I'll also include a few thoughts on practitioners you may choose to seek in your process. Good luck with your search for health and healing!

THINK

L. Hay (1984) *You Can Heal Your Life*. Carlsbad, CA: Hay House. This book, written many years ago, continues to hold one of my deepest beliefs: Most of us are ill because at some level we believe we're not good enough. Hay features conditions many of us express, then offers affirmations to help "heal" the condition.

L. Hay and M.L. Schulz (2014) *All Is Well*. New York: Hay House. In a much newer book, Louise Hay has teamed with researcher Mona Lisa Schulz to validate some of the ideas she propagated over the years about how emotions affect health... Schulz provides scientific evidence for many of Hay's claims.

N. Karrasch (2012) *Freeing Emotions and Energy through Myofascial Release*. London and Philadelphia: Singing Dragon. My second book, written primarily for bodyworkers but interesting to many clients, attempts to consolidate the models of Chinese medicine, the Indian chakra system, body psychology and myofascial release into one model to serve all healing.

L. Dossey (1995) *Healing Words: The Power of Prayer and the Practice of Medicine*. San Francisco: Harper. This scientist and neurosurgeon set out to prove prayer wasn't actually effective. Instead, in something like 115 studies, he found that 100 validated its effectiveness, and the most effective prayer is "Thy will be done."

J. Pierrakos (2005) *CORE Energetics*. Mendacino, CA: CORE Evolution. One of Wilhelm Reich's main disciples, Pierrakos theorizes that (in my interpretation) we are three-layered beings: the CORE is the Center Of Right Energy; the body, then the environment. Too many of us use our *bodies* to protect our *cores* from our *environment*.

J. Sarno (2006) *The Divided Mind*. London: Harper. Medical doctor Sarno suggests many of us suffer physically due to emotional issues from earlier times that haven't been released.

P. Levine (2010) *In an Unspoken Voice*. Berkeley, CA: North Atlantic Books. Levine, developer of Somatic Experiencing work, is a psychologist who suggests many of us choose to become trapped in our emotions and thus won't pay attention to our bodily sensations.

G. Enders (2015) *Gut: The Inside Story of Our Body's Most Under-Rated Organ*. Vancouver/Berkeley: Greystone Books. If you really want an intimate look at the workings of the digestive and eliminative systems and how important they are to health, this is the book.

Internet! While there is plenty of trash on the internet, there are also good sources. As with any source, take what you find with a dose of common sense, but don't discount internet searching when you have a situation that leads you to gather more information.

Emotional and Mental Therapies: Mental health is finally being recognized as an important aspect of overall health; these days, many insurance companies are finally respecting the need for mental health coverage. First rule: Do you feel safe with this practitioner? Do you feel you can absolutely share what needs to be shared? I'm not even sure we all need an outside practitioner, as much as a trusted friend who knows how to listen deeply, prod gently and validate thoroughly. Whether you consider psychotherapy, psychological counseling, Emotional Freedom Technique, Somatic Experiencing, Re-Evaluation counseling or any other type of mental stimulation, the question remains: Do you feel safe with this person?

ACT

P. Egoscue and R. Gittines (2000) *Pain Free: A Revolutionary Method for Stopping Chronic Pain*. New York: Random House. A very good book for serious seekers; while many of the exercises feel like nothing is happening, results can come. Warning! Don't overdo the work.

N. Karrasch (2009) *Meet Your Body: CORE Bodywork Tools to Release Bodymindcore Trauma*. London and Philadelphia: Singing Dragon. My first book designed to help clients realize there are hinges through the body; all of them need to be "oiled" through movement and awareness.

S. Rosenberg (2017) *Accessing the Healing Power of the Vagus Nerve*. Berkeley, CA: North Atlantic Books. I'm quite taken with Rosenberg's ideas explaining the vagus nerve and its functions and relationship to other nervous systems. He also offers easy-to-follow instructions for what I call a "vagal reset" and what he suggests is returning our body to a ventral vagal state instead of living in freeze, fight or flee. An important new book.

M. Bond (2007) *The New Rules of Posture.* Rochester, VT: Healing Arts Press. An earlier Mary Bond book; she has several, all good in terms of helping clients understand their bodies better and move them more effectively and happily.

B. Spindler (2018) *Yoga Therapy for Fear.* London and Philadelphia: Singing Dragon. My friend Beth Spindler has created a lovely book suggesting much of what keeps us from living our fullest life can be accessed and processed through simple yoga awareness.

Bodywork Therapies: There are many types of bodywork out there these days; nearly as many modalities as there are bodyworkers! I invite you to look for someone near you who offers the type of work that resonates; and I also invite you to make sure you feel safe and comfortable with this person and that you understand what they're trying to do with and for you, and how you can help them achieve your goals—*your* goals, not theirs. Be it Structural Integration, CORE Bodywork, deep tissue therapy, myofascial release, relaxation massage, shiatsu, Thai massage, etc, etc…the type of work is less important than the relationship you create with the practitioner. If their work makes sense to you and you feel you're a partner in the work, you're well on your way.

Movement Therapies: Again, there are so many different types of movement work, and the same rules apply! First, find someone you trust in a setting where you feel safe. Then make sure you understand what is being done and why. Remain your own authority; if something feels wrong to you, it probably is. Whether you pursue yoga, tai chi, chi gung, Pilates, body rolling or foam rolling, Alexander, Feldenkreis, Laban or any of the many types of movement therapies, like every other activity, what you put into it, and with what kind of dedication and expectation, will enhance your experience.

Index